COMPREHENSIVE

CLEFT CARE
Family Edition

COMPREHENSIVE
CLEFT CARE
Family Edition

Edited by

Joseph E. Losee, MD, FACS, FAAP
Ross H. Musgrave Professor of Pediatric Plastic Surgery;
Executive Vice-Chair and Program Director,
Department of Plastic Surgery,
University of Pittsburgh Medical Center;
Division Chief, Pediatric Plastic Surgery,
Children's Hospital of Pittsburgh of the University of Pittsburgh
Medical Center,
Pittsburgh, Pennsylvania

Richard E. Kirschner, MD, FACS, FAAP
Robert F. and Edgar T. Wolfe Foundation
Endowed Chair in Plastic and Reconstructive Surgery;
Chief, Section of Plastic and Reconstructive Surgery;
Director, Cleft Lip and Palate Center,
Nationwide Children's Hospital;
Professor of Surgery and Pediatrics,
Senior Vice Chair, Department of Plastic Surgery,
The Ohio State University College of Medicine,
Columbus, Ohio

Darren M. Smith, MD
Craniofacial Fellow,
Department of Plastic Surgery,
The Hospital for Sick Children,
Toronto, Ontario, Canada

With Co-editors

Christin R. Lawrence
Amy Straub

CRC CRC Press
Taylor & Francis Group
2015

CRC Press
Taylor & Francis Group
6000 Broken Sound Parkway NW, Suite 300
Boca Raton, FL 33487-2742

© 2015 by Taylor & Francis Group, LLC
CRC Press is an imprint of Taylor & Francis Group, an Informa business

No claim to original U.S. Government works

Printed on acid-free paper
Version Date: 20150220

International Standard Book Number-13: 978-1-4822-4368-0 (Paperback)

Visit the Taylor & Francis Web site at
http://www.taylorandfrancis.com

and the CRC Press Web site at
http://www.crcpress.com

For our patients and their families

EXECUTIVE EDITOR Sue Hodgson
SENIOR PROJECT EDITING MANAGER Carolyn Reich
SENIOR DEVELOPMENTAL EDITOR Megan Fennell
DEVELOPMENTAL EDITOR Lindsay Westbrook
GRAPHICS MANAGER Brett Stone
DIRECTOR OF ILLUSTRATION AND DESIGN Brenda Bunch
ILLUSTRATORS Amy D'Camp, Morgan Noonan, Christopher Smith
MANAGING EDITOR Suzanne Wakefield
MANUSCRIPT EDITOR Rebecca Sweeney
PROJECT MANAGER Kelly Mabie
PRODUCTION Chris Lane, Debra Clark
PROOFREADER Linda Maulin
INDEXER Nancy Newman

Contributors

Oluwaseun A. Adetayo, MD, FAAP
Assistant Professor, Division of Plastic Surgery, Albany Medical Center; Section Chief, Pediatric Plastic Surgery, The Bernard & Millie Duker Children's Hospital at Albany Medical Center, Albany, New York

Cassandra L. Aspinall, MSW, ACSW, LICSW
Clinical Assistant Professor, School of Social Work, University of Washington; Senior Social Worker, Social Work/Craniofacial Center, Seattle Children's Hospital, Seattle, Washington

Stephen B. Baker, MD, DDS, FACS
Professor and Program Director, Department of Plastic Surgery, MedStar Georgetown Hospital, Washington, DC; Medical Director, Craniofacial Anomalies Center, Plastic Surgery Department, Inova Children's Hospital, Falls Church, Virginia

Chelsea K. Bartley, BS
Graduate Student, Department of Communication Sciences and Disorders, University of Cincinnati, Cincinnati, Ohio

Osama A. Basri, BDS, MEd, FRCD(C)
Fellow, Cleft Craniofacial Orthodontics, Division of Pediatric Plastic Surgery, Children's Hospital of Pittsburgh of the University of Pittsburgh Medical Center, Pittsburgh, Pennsylvania

Adriane L. Baylis, PhD, CCC-SLP
Assistant Professor, Departments of Plastic Surgery, Pediatrics, and Speech and Hearing Science, The Ohio State University College of Medicine; Director, Velopharyngeal Dysfunction Program, Section of Plastic and Reconstructive Surgery, Nationwide Children's Hospital, Columbus, Ohio

Mary Breen, MS, RN
Clinical Nurse Specialist, Craniofacial and Reconstructive Plastic Surgery Center, Dell Children's Medical Center of Central Texas, Austin, Texas

Philip Kuo-Ting Chen, MD
Professor, Department of Plastic and Reconstructive Surgery, Chang Gung Memorial Hospital and Chang Gung University, Taipei, Taiwan

Patricia D. Chibbaro, RN, MS, CPNP
Pediatric Nurse Practitioner, Institute of Reconstructive Plastic Surgery, New York University Langone Medical Center, New York, New York

Franklyn P. Cladis, MD, FAAP
Associate Professor of Anesthesiology, Department of Anesthesiology, Children's Hospital of Pittsburgh of the University of Pittsburgh Medical Center, Pittsburgh, Pennsylvania

Marilyn A. Cohen, BA
Administrative Director and Patient Care Coordinator, Regional Cleft Palate-Craniofacial Program, Cooper University Hospital, Camden, New Jersey

Bernard J. Costello, DMD, MD
Professor and Program Director, Department of Oral and Maxillofacial Surgery, University of Pittsburgh School of Dental Medicine, Pittsburgh, Pennsylvania

Canice E. Crerand, PhD
Assistant Professor, Departments of Pediatrics and Plastic Surgery, The Ohio State University College of Medicine; Craniofacial Psychologist, Nationwide Children's Hospital, Columbus, Ohio

Michael L. Cunningham, MD, PhD
Professor, Department of Pediatrics, University of Washington; Program Director, Seattle Children's Craniofacial Center, Seattle Children's Hospital, Seattle, Washington

Donna Cutler-Landsman, MS
Retired Educator, Middleton-Cross Plains Area School District; Educational Consultant, Cutler-Landsman Consulting, Middleton, Wisconsin

Lauren DiCairano, BS
Clinic Coordinator, 22q and You Center, Department of Human Genetics, The Children's Hospital of Philadelphia, Philadelphia, Pennsylvania

Simone J. Fischbach, MHSc, SLP(C), Registered CASLPO
Lecturer, Department of Speech-Language Pathology, University of Toronto, Toronto, Ontario, Canada

Matthew D. Ford, MS, CCC-SLP
Clinical Coordinator, Cleft-Craniofacial Center, Children's Hospital of Pittsburgh of the University of Pittsburgh Medical Center, Pittsburgh, Pennsylvania

Christopher R. Forrest, MD, MSc, FRCSC, FACS
Chair, Division of Plastic and Reconstructive Surgery; Medical Director, Centre for Craniofacial Care and Research, The Hospital for Sick Children; Chair, Division of Plastic and Reconstructive Surgery, Department of Surgery, University of Toronto, Toronto, Ontario, Canada

Jesse A. Goldstein, MD
Assistant Professor of Surgery, Division of Pediatric Plastic Surgery, Children's Hospital of Pittsburgh of the University of Pittsburgh Medical Center; Assistant Professor, Department of Plastic Surgery, University of Pittsburgh Medical Center, Pittsburgh, Pennsylvania

Arun K. Gosain, MD
Professor and Chief, Division of Pediatric Plastic Surgery, Lurie Children's Hospital of Northwestern University Feinberg School of Medicine, Chicago, Illinois

Lynn Marty Grames, MA, CCC-SLP
Speech-Language Pathologist, Cleft Palate and Craniofacial Institute, St. Louis Children's Hospital; Adjunct Instructor, Department of Orthodontics, Department of Communication Sciences and Disorders, Saint Louis University, St. Louis, Missouri

Adelle Green
Volunteer, World Craniofacial Foundation, Dallas, Texas

Matthew Greives, MD
Assistant Professor, Department of Pediatric Surgery, Division of Pediatric Plastic Surgery, University of Texas Health Science Center at Houston, Houston, Texas

Jodi Gustave, MD
Department of Pulmonology, Nemours/Alfred I. duPont Hospital for Children, Wilmington, Delaware

Rachel Harmon, LICSW
Licensed Independent Clinical Social Worker, Pediatric Advanced Care Team, Seattle Children's Hospital, Seattle, Washington

Celia E. Heppner, PsyD
Assistant Professor, Department of Psychiatry, University of Texas Southwestern Medical School; Pediatric Psychologist, Fogelson Plastic and Craniofacial Surgery Center, Children's Health/Children's Medical Center Dallas, Dallas, Texas

Larry J. Hollier, MD
Chief, Department of Surgery, Division of Plastic Surgery, Baylor College of Medicine, Houston, Texas

Donald V. Huebener, DDS, MS, MAEd
Professor, Division of Plastic and Reconstructive Surgery, Washington University School of Medicine; Director of Pediatric Dentistry, St. Louis Children's Hospital, St. Louis, Missouri

Noel Jabbour, MD
Assistant Professor, Department of Otolaryngology, University of Pittsburgh School
of Medicine; Associate Fellowship Program Director; Director, Congenital Ear Center,
Department of Pediatric Otolaryngology, Children's Hospital of Pittsburgh of the University
of Pittsburgh Medical Center, Pittsburgh, Pennsylvania

Richard E. Kirschner, MD, FACS, FAAP
Robert F. and Edgar T. Wolfe Foundation Endowed Chair in Plastic and Reconstructive
Surgery; Chief, Section of Plastic and Reconstructive Surgery; Director, Cleft Lip and
Palate Center, Nationwide Children's Hospital; Professor of Surgery and Pediatrics, Senior
Vice Chair, Department of Plastic Surgery, The Ohio State University College of Medicine,
Columbus, Ohio

Paula G. Klaiman, MClSc, Reg. CASLPO
Lecturer, Department of Speech-Language Pathology, University of Toronto, Toronto,
Ontario, Canada

Ann W. Kummer, PhD, CCC-SLP, ASHA Fellow
Professor, Clinical Pediatrics and Otolaryngology Department, University of Cincinnati
College of Medicine; Senior Director, Division of Speech-Language Pathology, Cincinnati
Children's Hospital Medical Center, Cincinnati, Ohio

Steven T. Lanier, MD
Division of Plastic Surgery, Northwestern University Feinberg School of Medicine, Chicago,
Illinois

Christin R. Lawrence
Parent, Westerville, Ohio

Dawn Leavitt, RN-BC, BSN
Nurse Clinician Care Coordinator, Craniofacial Center, Seattle Children's Hospital, Seattle,
Washington

Joseph E. Losee, MD, FACS, FAAP
Ross H. Musgrave Professor of Pediatric Plastic Surgery; Executive Vice-Chair and Program
Director, Department of Plastic Surgery, University of Pittsburgh Medical Center; Division
Chief, Pediatric Plastic Surgery, Children's Hospital of Pittsburgh of the University of
Pittsburgh Medical Center, Pittsburgh, Pennsylvania

Donna M. McDonald-McGinn, MS, LGC
Clinical Professor of Pediatrics, Department of Pediatrics, The Perelman School of Medicine
of the University of Pennsylvania; Associate Director, Clinical Genetics Center; Director, 22q
and You Center; Chief, Section of Genetic Counseling; Department of Human Genetics, The
Children's Hospital of Philadelphia, Philadelphia, Pennsylvania

Michael Mennuti, MD, FACOG, FACMG
William Goodell Professor of Obstetrics and Gynecology, Department of Obstetrics and Gynecology, University of Pennsylvania, Philadelphia, Pennsylvania

Ana M. Mercado, DMD, MS, PhD
Clinical Assistant Professor, Department of Orthodontics, The Ohio State University College of Dentistry; Member of Medical Staff, Department of Orthodontics, Nationwide Children's Hospital, Columbus, Ohio

Laura A. Monson, MD
Assistant Professor, Department of Surgery, Division of Plastic Surgery, Baylor College of Medicine, Houston, Texas

Mark P. Mooney, PhD
Professor and Chair, Department of Oral Biology, School of Dental Medicine; Professor, Departments of Anthropology, Plastic Surgery, Orthodontics, and Communication and Speech Disorders, and Cleft Palate-Craniofacial Center, University of Pittsburgh, Pittsburgh, Pennsylvania

Gregory D. Pearson, MD, FACS, FAAP
Assistant Professor of Clinical Plastic Surgery, Department of Plastic Surgery, The Ohio State University; Director, Center for Complex Craniofacial Disorders, Nationwide Children's Hospital, Columbus, Ohio

Barry L. Ramsey, BS
Research Associate, UNC Center for Health Promotion and Disease Prevention, University of North Carolina at Chapel Hill, Chapel Hill, North Carolina

Ramon L. Ruiz, DMD, MD
Associate Professor of Surgery, University of Central Florida College of Medicine; Director, Pediatric Craniomaxillofacial Surgery; Vice Chair, Department of Surgery, Arnold Palmer Hospital for Children, Orlando, Florida

Diane L. Sabo, PhD
Associate Professor, Department of Communication Science and Disorders, School of Health and Rehabilitation Sciences, University of Pittsburgh, Pittsburgh, Pennsylvania

Susan M. Salkowitz, MA, MGA
Adjunct Senior Fellow, Leonard Davis Institute of Health Economics, University of Pennsylvania, Philadelphia, Pennsylvania

Ashley Salyer
Volunteer, World Craniofacial Foundation, Dallas, Texas

Kenneth E. Salyer, MD, FACS, FAAP
Clinical Professor, Department of Biomedical Sciences; Adjunct Professor, Department of Orthodontics, Texas A&M University, Baylor College of Dentistry, Dallas, Texas

Lindsay A. Schuster, DMD, MS
Clinical Assistant Professor of Plastic Surgery, Department of Plastic Surgery, University of Pittsburgh; Director, Cleft-Craniofacial Orthodontics, Children's Hospital of Pittsburgh of the University of Pittsburgh Medical Center, Pittsburgh, Pennsylvania

E. Gail Shaffer, MD, MPH
Anesthesiologist, General Anesthesia Services, Inc., Charleston, West Virginia

Darren M. Smith, MD
Craniofacial Fellow, Department of Plastic Surgery, The Hospital for Sick Children, Toronto, Ontario, Canada

Kelsey Smith, MS, CGC
Certified Genetic Counselor, Department of Clinical Genetics, Children's Hospital of Philadelphia, Philadelphia, Pennsylvania

Mark Splaingard, MD
Professor, Pediatrics Department, Ohio State Medical School; Director of Pediatric Sleep Center, Nationwide Children's Hospital, Columbus, Ohio

Amy Straub, MA, CCC-SLP
Parent, St. Marys, Pennsylvania

Ronald P. Strauss, DMD, PhD
Executive Vice Provost and Chief International Officer; Professor, Social Medicine, University of North Carolina at Chapel Hill, Chapel Hill, North Carolina

Stephanie E. Watkins, PhD, MSPH, MSPT
Postdoctoral Research Fellow, UNC Center for Health Promotion and Disease Prevention, University of North Carolina at Chapel Hill, Chapel Hill, North Carolina

Preface

Professionals have long recognized that the best cleft care is team care. Although most parents think of a clinical care team as one comprising a group of medical providers, the simple truth is that families and other caregivers play an equally important role in ensuring that a child born with a cleft lip/palate enjoys the greatest possible quality of life.

This book was written to provide families with the information necessary to fully understand their child's condition, its consequences, and its treatment. It is our hope that this edition will serve as an effective tool that will enable parents and families to play a central role in navigating their child's care journey, working alongside the rest of the team to ensure that their child has every opportunity to reach his or her full potential.

Joseph E. Losee
Richard E. Kirschner
Darren M. Smith

Acknowledgments

As is the finest cleft care, this book was truly a team effort. We would like to acknowledge the excellent contributions of the authors who shared their expertise in the chapters of *Family Edition;* they have graciously provided their insights in creating this important resource for parents of cleft-affected children.

We also acknowledge the teachers and mentors who have challenged us, inspired us, and who, in profound ways, have shaped our vision and our working lives. We are grateful as well to our wonderful patients and their families who have challenged and inspired us in their own way. We thank our own families for their support and patience as we navigated the challenges of completing both the second edition of *Comprehensive Cleft Care* and this new work. To our teams, we owe a debt of gratitude for their tireless efforts; whatever the task, they find a way to get it done with excellence.

Our sincere thanks are due to the creative team at CRC Press, Taylor & Francis Group, for producing this work. Executive Editor Sue Hodgson, Senior Developmental Editor Megan Fennell, and Developmental Editor Lindsay Westbrook kept us on track in drafting, assembling, and transmitting well-crafted chapters. A group of illustrators, headed by Brenda Bunch, rendered the beautiful drawings throughout, and layout artist Debra Clark composed the text and images into a coherent, reader-friendly whole. Editor Rebecca Sweeney polished our paragraphs, and Project Manager Kelly Mabie guided us through the page review stages. Team leaders Carolyn Reich and Brett Stone worked their magic in ensuring the clear, elegant graphics and layout for which this team is known.

And we offer our deepest appreciation to Christin Lawrence and Amy Straub, both knowledgeable, devoted parents of cleft-affected children, who reviewed every chapter and contributed their own insights. These parent-editors helped to ensure that *Family Edition* provides the sound, accessible information that parents and family need to feel empowered to make appropriate care decisions for their children, to feel comfortable asking questions, and to face the challenges and successes of their children's care and treatment.

Introduction

This book is supplemental to the professional textbook *Comprehensive Cleft Care*, second edition. The *Family Edition* is a comprehensive guide on cleft lip and palate, written largely in language that parents of cleft-affected children can easily understand. This book is an invaluable resource for families and is the only one of its kind published to date.

When asked to co-edit this parent's guide, we were both thrilled to have been chosen to be a part of this important project, and we were thankful to contribute out of a framework of personal experience, since we are parents of cleft-affected children.

Although we have traveled different paths with our cleft-affected children, we both have committed ourselves to obtaining the best treatment possible for them. Amy did not know that her son had a unilateral cleft lip and palate until he was born. Christin and her husband adopted their daughter internationally and were aware of her unilateral cleft lip and palate before bringing her home.

We both found excellent medical doctors and teams who helped us in shaping a plan for the best outcomes for our children. However, even while receiving wonderful care from the medical professionals, there were often many unanswered questions and concerns. We agree that had we had a parent's guide such as the *Family Edition* in our hands, many of our anxieties about what to expect regarding our children's care would have been alleviated, even if just to help us as parents feel more educated and empowered, by having the information at our disposal at home (where most parents try to remember all that the doctors said at the last appointment).

Our own children have come far in their journeys, but they are also far from the end. We understand the stress and anxiety that come with each recommendation for another treatment or surgical procedure. We have tried to assist the authors of the *Family Edition* by reading their writings from a parent's perspective to make certain that the information provided is not only informative and helpful but also readily accessible and as relevant as possible. It was very important to us that any parent could use this guide without difficulty.

We have had the opportunity to read the work of some of the most outstanding professionals from some of the best cleft teams in the country, and they welcomed our suggestions and edits. Our hope is that you find this a helpful reference guide throughout your child's process of care and treatment.

As you embark on this journey with your child, there may be many challenges, unexpected disappointments, and successes along the way. Having a reference to use to help reduce some of the stress associated with raising a cleft-affected child will only enhance your ability to care for your child.

Whether you have recently found out that you are expecting and are just beginning to research your child's diagnosis, or whether your child is older and is continuing with treatments, know that we are both honored and humbled to have contributed to your lives in some small way, and wish you and your family the best.

Christin R. Lawrence
Amy Straub

Contents

Part IV Airway and Breathing Issues

Part V Cleft Lip and Palate Repair

Part VI Cleft Palate Dental and Orthodontic Principles

Part I

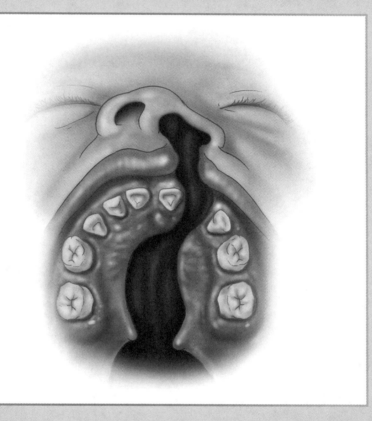

Fundamentals of Cleft Care

Fundamentals of Team Care

Marilyn A. Cohen

KEY POINTS

○ Team care is the highest standard of care for patients with craniofacial differences.

○ Team care saves patients and families time and money.

○ The patient and family are important members of the team.

○ Teams differ by type, members, mission, and procedures.

○ Cleft palate teams specifically serve patients who have a cleft of the lip or palate.

○ Craniofacial teams serve patients who have other differences of the skull, jaws, or face. At some centers, this team also sees patients who have a cleft of the lip or palate.

A craniofacial team is the best option for providing care to a patient with a *craniofacial* condition. A craniofacial team is a group of doctors and other medical professionals who care for patients with conditions of the skull and/or face. A *cleft palate* team is a type of craniofacial team that focuses on patients with a cleft lip or palate. These types of teams have been serving children in the United States since 1938. Doctors and patients know how important it is to coordinate the many different types of care needed by children with cleft palate and other craniofacial differences. Today there are more than 250 cleft palate and/or craniofacial teams in the United States and Canada, with new teams continuing to form around the world.

A craniofacial team brings many specialists together to evaluate the specific needs of each patient and to prioritize and schedule services to meet these needs. Craniofacial differences affect many aspects of a patient's life. Depending on the patient's needs, the team may include the services of many specialists such as the following:
- *Audiologist*
- Dentist
- Feeding specialist
- Geneticist/genetic counselor
- Neurosurgeon
- Nurse/nurse practitioner
- *Ophthalmologist*
- *Oral surgeon*
- Orthodontist
- *Otolaryngologist*
- Pediatrician
- *Plastic surgeon*
- *Psychologist*
- *Social worker*
- *Speech-language pathologist*
- Other medical professionals

BENEFITS OF TEAM CARE

Team care has many benefits. The most important benefit is that team members work together to address the patient's needs; they share their findings so that each health care provider has an overview of a patient's condition and needs rather than one single view. The team then creates one comprehensive and coordinated treatment plan. For example, the patient's physical condition may be the most obvious issue; however, the team can plan for guidance to help the patient and family deal with teasing and/or bullying. They might group multiple procedures into one surgery. Specific members of the team can provide braces for the patient's teeth, if needed, and others offer counseling to cope with feelings about looking different. Some patients need help with school issues. A family may need financial or transportation assistance. The team considers all of the patient's and family's needs.

In addition, team visits save the patient and family time and money. Team visits often last a half-day or a full day, much longer than an average doctor's visit.

However, during that time, the patient sees specialists at only one location. With team care, families spend less time overall at doctors' offices, leaving more time for their own activities. Overall, team care provides the patient and family with an effective way to access care.

Characteristics of Team Care

Differences Between Cleft Palate and Craniofacial Teams

Most craniofacial teams in the United States are made up of members who belong to the American Cleft Palate-Craniofacial Association (ACPA), an organization that sets the standards for team care. Cleft palate teams and craniofacial teams are the two types of teams that treat children with craniofacial differences. They differ by the patients they see and the members of their teams.

A cleft palate team usually sees patients with clefts of the lip and palate. These teams also often see patients with *velopharyngeal dysfunction,* or hypernasal speech, but who do not have a cleft palate. Cleft palate teams typically include the following medical providers:

- Patient care coordinator (who makes appointments and helps to arrange for the patient's care)
- Speech-language pathologist (speech therapist)
- Orthodontist
- Surgeon

Each of these team members has special training in treating cleft palate patients. These teams also consult with professionals in the following fields:

- Audiology
- Dentistry
- Genetics
- Otolaryngology
- Pediatrics or primary care
- Psychiatry
- Psychology
- Social work

The second type of team is a craniofacial team. This team sees patients with more complex craniofacial issues; in some centers, they also see patients with clefts of the lip and/or palate. Craniofacial teams include the same providers described previously plus additional members with special training. The team's surgeon has special training in surgery of the head, neck, face, jaw, and mouth. This type of surgery is known as *craniomaxillofacial surgery.* The psychologist working with a craniofacial team has training in testing learning skills and intelligence through psychoeducational testing. The psychologist tests emotional state and social relationships through psychosocial testing. Some teams perform neuropsychological testing. These tests evaluate intelligence, attention, memory, small motor skills, large motor skills, self-control, and more. The craniofacial team may include, or may provide direct referrals to, the following specialists:

- *Geneticist*
- Neurosurgeon
- Ophthalmologist
- Radiologist

Team Functioning

Teams differ by more than their type of team or their members' specialties. They also differ in the way they function. Teams can be multidisciplinary, transdisciplinary, or interdisciplinary.

On multidisciplinary teams, each team member provides care strictly within his or her expertise. Each team member examines the patient. Team members then compare notes through meetings, emails, or written reports. Next, the team combines all the separate findings and creates a list of recommendations.

On transdisciplinary teams, team members learn about each other's fields of expertise. This blurs the boundaries between professions. In addition, team members' professional roles may change from patient to patient. For example, the dentist might ask questions about speech, and the psychologist might ask questions about teeth. These team members often share information with each other in a less formal way.

Interdisciplinary teams have features of the other two types of teams. The roles of the members overlap somewhat, but not as much as on transdisciplinary teams. Overlap occurs when more than one team member examines the same body part or skill. For example, the dentist may discuss how tooth position can affect speech. The speech-language pathologist may recommend a specific surgery for speech. Team members share their findings with each other formally or informally. Most craniofacial teams are interdisciplinary. This team model works well for craniofacial and cleft palate teams for two reasons. First, it supports equal contributions from all team members. Second, it promotes problem-solving that involves all team members.

Team Mission

Teams may also differ in their mission. A team's mission is a description of its goals. These goals might address patient care, research, public service, or education. Their purpose is to affect and improve patient care in the short and long term. Team missions often differ according to the location of the team. Teams in universities or teaching hospitals often have research and education goals. On the other hand, patient care is sometimes the only focus for teams in medical centers or private clinics.

Each type of mission has many benefits. For instance, teams involved in research may offer the newest techniques. The patient may have the option to participate in studies that can improve care for all. In teaching hospitals or universities, students and research assistants may take part in the team visit. Some patients are overwhelmed by the number of people involved in their care. Other patients enjoy having more people involved. Most teams will include their mission on their website or in their welcome packets. For examples of team missions, see Table 1-1.

Table 1-1   Examples of Team Missions

University-Based Team	Hospital-Based Team
"The mission of the UNCCFC is to provide optimal care for patients with cleft lip, cleft palate, and other craniofacial anomalies through an interdisciplinary team-oriented approach and to stimulate biological, behavioral, and clinical research that will ultimately lead to an improved quality of life for our patients."*	"The mission of the Regional Craniofacial Center at St. Joseph's Children's Hospital is to provide quality specialized team care to children and adolescents with clefts and other congenital and/or acquired craniofacial anomalies. At St. Joseph's Regional Craniofacial Center, a premier multidisciplinary team of pediatric specialists provides consultation, diagnosis, and treatment for patients with craniofacial disorders as well as education and support for their family members."†

*From the University of North Carolina Craniofacial Team website, 2014.
†From St. Joseph's Regional Craniofacial Center website, 2014.
UNCCFC, University of North Carolina Craniofacial Center.

The Team Visit

Each team has its own method of conducting a team visit. Most team visits take approximately half a day for the patient and family. However, some may take a full day, depending on the team's schedule. Most team visits begin with a discussion with the patient care coordinator. Family members are often asked to complete a clinical questionnaire and insurance forms. They will also fill out release-of-information forms. These forms allow the team to talk with the patient's doctors, therapists, and teachers. The family pays any required copays or other fees. Many teams give the family a packet describing the team members and a schedule for the day. Some teams regularly take pictures of the patient to maintain a visual record of the patient over time.

Although the details of the team visit will vary from team to team, three types of team visits are most common.

In the first type of team visit (Fig. 1-1), patients and families wait in one or more waiting rooms. Some clinics are set up in one suite of offices where all the team members see the patients. Other clinics have waiting rooms in a few different areas. In other cases, groups of team members may be located in different parts of the hospital. The patient care coordinator often guides patients and families between these waiting rooms.

One by one, each team member takes the patient and family to his or her office for an evaluation. Sometimes several team members will see the patient together, depending on the patient's needs, scheduling issues, and space limitations.

At the end of each team member's evaluation, the patient returns to the waiting room. The patient then waits to be seen by the next team member. Each of these evaluations will vary from a few minutes to an hour or more. The amount of time depends on the patient's needs and age.

In another type of team visit (Fig. 1-2), patients and families wait in a treatment room. The team members come in one-by-one to evaluate the patient in one room. The patient and family remain together. The patient may not see every team member every year. This depends on the patient's age. For example, very young children may not see the *orthodontist* until they are a bit older.

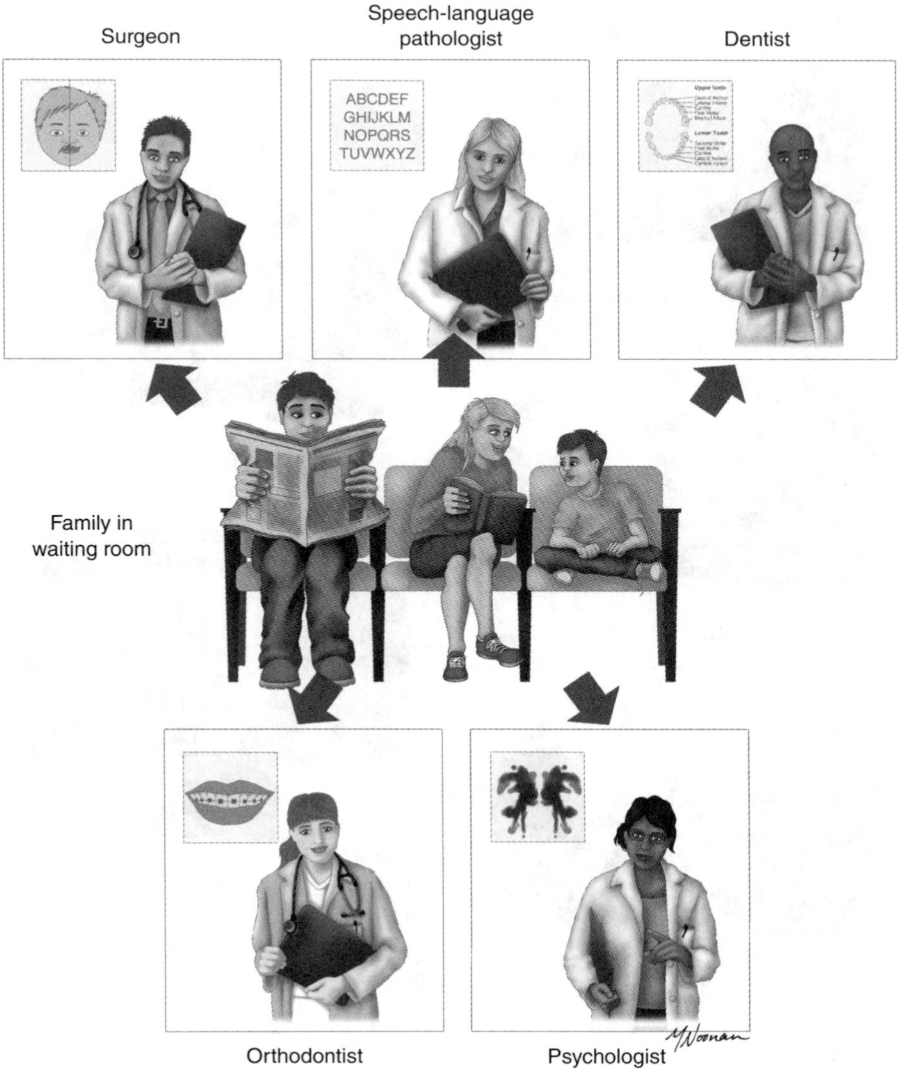

Fig. 1-1   Team visit type 1. The family moves from the waiting room to the examination rooms.

Family in examination room

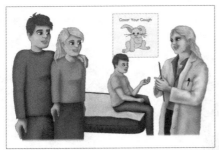

Speech-language pathologist

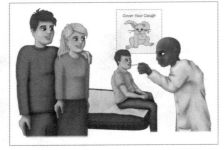

Dentist

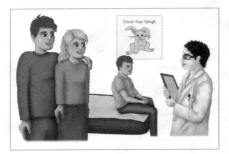

Surgeon

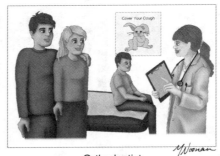

Orthodontist

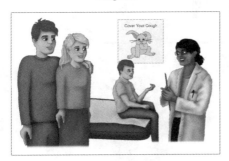

Psychologist

Fig. 1-2   Team visit type 2. The team providers move, while the patient and family stay in the examination room.

The third type of visit is a less common type of craniofacial team visit (Fig. 1-3). The patient and family remain in an observation room instead of a waiting room or treatment room. One or two team members complete all parts of the team evaluation. The other team members watch and evaluate, either in the same room as the patient or behind one-way mirrors. This arena-style visit is more common with transdisciplinary teams.

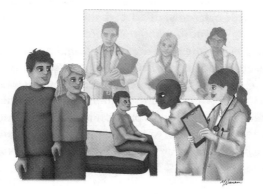

Fig. 1-3   Team visit type 3. The patient is examined by two team members while the rest of the team observes.

Most teams schedule visits on a yearly basis. However, some patients may have a more pressing need that requires another visit in less than a year. At other times, patients may have no need to return in the coming year and may then be scheduled to return in 2 years or more.

The Team Meeting

At the end of each team visit, all of the information about the patient is gathered together for review. The team then decides which procedures or treatments the patient requires. Next, the team develops a plan and a treatment schedule to best meet the patient's needs. Most teams send patients home before the team meeting to await the team's written recommendations. Some teams have a team member explain the treatment plan to the family after the team meeting. Other teams will invite the family to take part in the team meeting and to be present while the team discusses all of the options.

The purpose of the team meeting is to create a treatment plan for the patient. This plan addresses the child's medical, psychosocial, and educational needs. The team will usually send this plan in a written report to the family through the mail. It is the family's responsibility to follow through with the recommendations. The patient care coordinator will help the family set up some of the appointments. If possible, more than one appointment will be scheduled on the same day to save time and travel expenses. The team sends the report to the health care providers selected by the family. The patient's community health care providers will need the team report to plan the best treatment. In turn, the team needs information from the patient's doctors, teachers, and therapists. These reports show the patient's progress and needs from year to year.

The team meeting is one of the most important team functions. A well-run team will make the most current and effective recommendations for patient care. The team will also help to decide the best order for carrying out these recommendations. They will try to schedule some surgical procedures together. For example, the patient may need to have ear tubes placed and a surgical procedure to correct speech. Without a team, the patient would likely have two separate surgeries. Team surgeons work together to take care of as many of the patient's needs as possible during one operation.

The Patient and Family as Team Members

The patient and family are among the most important team members. After all, the focus of the team is the patient's and family's needs. As patients grow and mature, their role on the team will change. When patients are very young, the focus is on what the parents and professionals think is required. As patients mature and become more aware of personal wants and needs, they become more involved in making decisions about their own care. As active team members, patients and parents have the following responsibilities:
- Provide the team with as much information as possible.
- Send school and medical records to the team.
- Tell the team about the patient's and family's most important concerns.
- Tell the team when the family does not agree with the team's recommendations.
- Tell the team when the family cannot carry out the team's recommendations.
- Make and keep appointments throughout the year.
- Follow through with recommendations for home such as:
  - Massaging scars
  - Practicing speech exercises
  - Brushing teeth

The number of doctor visits and treatments can be overwhelming for patients and their families. Other commitments can make it hard to follow team recommendations. Cost and/or insurance issues may limit what the family can do. These are important matters to discuss with the team. Knowledge of any family issues is important when creating a patient care plan. The team can often provide the following assistance:
- Help the family find local agencies:
  - Transportation
  - Medicaid

  - Financial help
  - Respite care
- Help the family find local professionals:
  - Dentists
  - Doctors
  - Orthodontists
  - Therapists based in schools or private practice
- Help to advocate for needed services in school

Sometimes the patient has problems that need to be resolved quickly to prevent larger issues. In these rare cases, the team works with the family to ensure that the patient receives needed care as soon as possible.

Choosing a Team

When a child is born with a craniofacial difference, the birth hospital often refers the patient to a local team. Some families, however, do not have this help in finding care for their child. In either case, the family may wish to learn more about the team or teams in their area. Larger cities might have several teams. In rural areas, it can be difficult to find team care that is close to home. Some families will ask friends and family members if they know of any doctors or teams. Many families will use the Internet to search for what they need. Internet users should be aware that not all information on the web is correct. The Cleft Palate Foundation (*www. cleftline.org;* 1-800-24-CLEFT) serves as a trusted source for parents seeking information. Parents can call or search their website for a credentialed cleft palate or craniofacial team in their area. Families can also find answers to their questions about craniofacial conditions.

Teams differ in size, types of providers, and experience. Some teams see patients on a weekly basis. Other teams see patients monthly or only a few times a year. Teams that see more patients usually have more experience with the care that patients need. Some only have the basic cleft palate team members: a surgeon, an orthodontist, and a speech-language pathologist. Most teams, however, include other medical providers who may be needed to provide comprehensive care.

Patients and parents choose teams for many different reasons. Some families select the team recommended by the birth hospital. Others choose a team by its location. Still others travel farther because of a team's reputation. Some families prefer to go to a small group of professionals. Others would rather have many specialists available for their child.

Families may also consider the type of evaluation a team uses when they choose a team. Some families prefer to see each individual team member. Others prefer the arena model in which they meet with only one or two team members.

In many parts of the country, only one team is available in a region. Some families will opt to travel to see distant teams. Not many families, however, have the time or resources for this option. Military families often have to move away from their established team. Some of these families have the option to travel back to their original team. Regardless of which team cares for the patient, team care is the highest standard of care for patients with cleft and craniofacial conditions. Studies show that patients cared for by craniofacial teams have better outcomes than those who go to independent medical providers.

TIMELINE FOR TEAM VISITS

- The infant is identified with a craniofacial condition, sometimes at birth and sometimes in later childhood.
- The patient and family attend team meetings every 1 to 3 years, depending on the patient's needs.
- The patient is discharged from the team's care once major care is completed. This usually occurs when the patient is 18 to 21 years of age.
- Some patients will seek team care as adults should the need arise.

CONCLUSION

Craniofacial team care is considered the highest standard of care for patients with cleft and craniofacial conditions. Evaluating all aspects of the patient at one time allows the team to address all of the patient's needs. Teams will differ by their team members, their mission, how they function, and how they run their team visit. However, the patient and family are key members of any cleft or craniofacial team, and their contributions help to direct and improve team outcomes. Outcomes improve most when patients and family members express their needs and carry out team recommendations. Patient outcomes are better with team care than with care from individual providers.

2

Advocacy for Cleft-Affected Children

Marilyn A. Cohen, Susan M. Salkowitz

KEY POINTS

○ Advocacy must be distinguished from lobbying, which is prohibited by the bylaws of many professional organizations.

○ Patients, families, and health care providers are responsible for advocating to ensure the continued availability of cleft care and funding mechanisms.

○ Government-based health care funding is regulated at the state and federal level. An understanding of these systems is helpful in planning successful advocacy strategies.

○ Advocacy efforts are dramatically enhanced by cooperation between families of cleft-affected children and their health care providers.

The Merriam-Webster dictionary defines the word advocate as one who supports or promotes the interests of another. A lobbyist is one who influences or sways someone toward a desired action. The manner in which a person or group supports and promotes the interest of another often determines whether they are lobbying or advocating for a specific cause or condition. These words have specific legal definitions. The right to lobby rather than advocate is often determined by the articles of incorporation of the institution or organization represented. The articles of incorporation of most 501(c)(3) nonprofit organizations are written in such a way that lobbying is essentially forbidden, but advocacy in the form of public education is within the scope of the bylaws. The American Cleft Palate-Craniofacial Association provides an excellent example in Article XIII of its bylaws, Activities of the Association. It states "the association shall not participate or intervene in . . . any political campaign on behalf of any candidate for public office." Therefore using the powers of the association to influence the election of a specific candidate would violate the bylaw, as would the donation of money in the name of the association to the campaigns of specific legislators who might support a health care bill. The Cleft Palate Foundation has a similar clause related to lobbying but states in the preamble to its bylaws that it is acceptable to facilitate and encourage the care of affected individuals. In this example, testifying before the legislature for continued support for the funding of cleft-craniofacial programs would be an acceptable form of advocacy and not considered lobbying.

Advocating for individuals with cleft and craniofacial conditions can be multifaceted. It can relate to direct patient care (for example, explaining to a school board the importance of continuing speech therapy through high school, or explaining to an insurance company why a given procedure is medically necessary and not simply cosmetic) and to the accessibility of services (for example, patients and/or parents reinforcing the value of the cleft-craniofacial team to hospital administrators to help a program retain its level of care). External pressure from the consumers of health care in today's environment does a great deal to ensure the viability of special programs.

Advocacy and lobbying are related concepts but are separated by focus. Advocates support or promote the interests of others; lobbyists attempt to convince others with particular interests to complete a specific action. The articles of incorporation of most 501(c)(3) nonprofit organizations are written to essentially forbid lobbying but to allow advocacy in the form of public education. Advocacy in the health care environment has become integral to the care of patients with special health care needs. Without the education provided by the consumers of services and the organizations representing those who provide care, it is unlikely that the passage of health care legislation and regulation to aid these patients, such as rules governing the coverage of preexisting conditions by insurance carriers, could have occurred.

The public and professional education provided by consumers and providers of cleft-craniofacial care have helped to shape the provision of care in the United States since the 1930s. This is exemplified by the passage of the federal Maternal and Child Health Act and the extension of Social Security benefits for those affected by handicapping conditions. Both acts allow most children in the United States to receive basic cleft care regardless of their family's ability to pay for it. Consumers of health care for special needs should consider legislators as a part of their health care team and correspond with them on health care issues. Almost every state in the United States posts a legislative roster comprising lists of legislative committee members assigned to specific programs such as insurance, education, and welfare. The United States federal legislature posts its own legislative roster. Members of Congress, whether at the state level or the federal level, vote to represent the interests of their constituents; therefore the voice of the consumer is of paramount importance.

HISTORY OF MATERNAL AND CHILD HEALTH SERVICES IN THE UNITED STATES

The crash of the stock market in 1929 resulted in a major decline in income and the ability of many families to provide basic nutrition and medical care for their children, especially those affected by infantile paralysis and other crippling conditions. Legislation passed in the 1930s enacted aid to dependent women and children, including care from established prenatal clinics and basic nutrition. It eased the burden on families caring for children with polio. Known in many states in the 1930s as the Crippled Children's Act, this legislation formed the basis of today's federal Title V Maternal and Child Health Program, one of the subsidies available for children with special health care needs. The Maternal and Child Health Program was modified in the 1980s into a block grant, which has become a match of federal and state monies. However, the allocation method for this money for the care of children with clefts and craniofacial conditions is determined by the department of health in each state. Title V funds are known as "last dollar funding"; they can only be accessed after all other third-party funding resources, including Medicaid, are exhausted. Although the federal government sets the parameters for last dollar spending and targets specific initiatives that must be addressed in the states' funding plans for this money, the allocation of the funds for these initiatives is state dependent. However, access to this money by an individual state requires the state to submit a comprehensive spending plan to the federal government every 5 years, with annual updates addressing the federal initiatives.

The use of this money for direct patient care and the process by which those with cleft and craniofacial conditions can obtain this money is unique in each state. Because Title V programs are funded through a federal block grant with a state match and must be reapplied for every 5 years, vigilance on the part of the consumer and the providers of health care is needed.

Most states annually review the health priorities addressed by the Maternal and Child Health Program block grant at a public hearing. At the time of these reviews, public comment is sought regarding the initiatives addressed and those not addressed adequately. Consumers and providers of the services outlined in these plans are encouraged to give both oral and written testimony. A lack of comments in some states has resulted in language specific to orofacial clefts and craniofacial conditions being removed from the health plan and replaced with more generic language such as "children with special health care needs." This can potentially place one childhood problem in competition for funding with another.

The state of Pennsylvania was once a model for the provision and funding of services related to cleft care because of the dedication and persistence of Dr. Robert Ivy and Dr. Herbert Cooper in the 1950s. Dr. Cooper, an orthodontist, founded the first interdisciplinary clinic for cleft care, the Lancaster Cleft Palate Clinic. He and Dr. Ivy, a surgeon, spent a good deal of time educating Pennsylvania legislators about the comprehensive care needed for children with clefts and craniofacial conditions and explaining that without appropriate interdisciplinary care, a cleft can be a handicapping condition. The education provided to the legislature by these doctors resulted in coverage for care and a dedicated oversight program for this care under maternal and child health services. The cleft program in Pennsylvania continued for decades, and its viability was eventually taken for granted. Lack of vigilance by care providers in the late 1990s and early 2000s resulted in the loss of specific language and funding related to cleft and craniofacial care.

Providers and consumers of services for children with special health care needs can take an active role in educating legislators and public health officials on the needs of children with clefts and craniofacial conditions by submitting testimony when maternal and child health plans are reviewed at the state level. The public hearing dates for these plans can be found on the Department of Health website for each state. Plans are generally reviewed in the spring of the year, and public comment is welcome.

SUPPLEMENTAL SOCIAL SECURITY INCOME

Those with specific types of disability may be ineligible for supplemental income through Social Security assistance and state Medicaid funds. The ability of a person with a cleft or craniofacial condition to receive any of these funds is dependent on an application process that rates the disability and family income. Families with members affected by a craniofacial condition, especially those with conditions requiring a great deal of medical and custodial intervention, should apply for supplemental income. Applications can be made through a local Social Security office.

INSURANCE LEGISLATION AND HEALTH CARE

Although federal legislation exists for health insurance and the requirements for basic coverage, many commercial group insurance plans are generally regulated by the state rather than the federal government. The regulation of commercial group insurance plans is entirely state dependent; therefore regional differences may occur regarding what is and is not covered relative to cleft craniofacial care. Many states, for example, have legislation relating to the need to cover all aspects of cleft or craniofacial care, including dental care and, in some instances, hearing aids and related appliances. However, in most instances, regulations only apply to group insurance plans written by commercial insurers. The insurance commissioner in the state usually has jurisdiction over such plans, and after review of an insurance denial can mandate that the commercial insurer cover a procedure. The problem is that many insurance providers or third-party payers operate outside of the jurisdiction of the insurance commissioner and state-specific legislation because the insurance plan is either a self-insured or managed-care plan. Many businesses self-insure their employees, and many trade unions underwrite insurance through their health and welfare plans. Self-insurance plans are not regulated by state legislation, but rather are federally regulated. Businesses that self-insure their employees must provide plans that have minimum benefits under the Employee Retirement Income Security Act of 1974 and the Affordable Health Care Act. Union health and welfare insurance plans are governed by the Department of Labor, and the review of an insurance denial relative to these plans has multiple layers. When appeals are needed for either a self-insurance plan or a union-based plan, the starting point after the required appeal process by the insurer is the employee's human resource or personnel department at their place of employment. The regulation and appeal process varies by state. Regulation in New Jersey, for example, is administered by the Department of Health, whereas regulation in other states may be under the Division of Banking and Insurance. The best resource for information on all insurance issues is the office of the state's insurance commissioner. This department can direct inquirers to appropriate regulating resources for information on appeals.

SPECIAL HEALTH NEEDS AND PUBLIC EDUCATION

Not all children with a cleft and/or craniofacial condition require a specialized educational environment; however, some may require special educational and or school-based therapeutic services. In the 1970s federal law was enacted governing the education of all children with handicapping conditions, widening the scope of services provided by a school district. This was originally known as Public Law

94-142 and was later renamed the Individuals With Disabilities Education Act. The law mandated that all states make available to children with disabilities a free and appropriate education in the least-restrictive environment. This law established procedures by which children with disabilities should be evaluated and classified to provide them with appropriate individualized education programs, known as IEPs. The law ensured that all IEPs be jointly developed between parents and school officials.

Because all states are federally mandated to provide specialized education, the process of obtaining special education is similar in all states and is related to due process of the law. In addition to education starting at the first grade level, most states have early-intervention programs for children with developmental delay from birth to 3 years of age. Obtaining information about programs for children under 3 years of age is best done by contacting the state's Division of Mental Health. For children from 3 to 6 years of age who need special educational services, information can usually be obtained through the local school district. The local school district can then refer families to the appropriate resource for continued educational testing and support. Other programs known as 504 plans are available within local school districts to provide monitoring for children with special needs who do not require an IEP but who do need occasional monitoring of their progress. An example of a 504 plan is the monitoring of a child with a developmental speech problem who currently does not need therapy but who might require therapy in the future. Another example of a 504 plan is one that provides special accommodations for a child with an attention deficit hyperactivity disorder during testing situations, when a special educational program is otherwise unnecessary. The local school district should be able to direct a family to appropriate resources for this accommodation, such as a child study team or a school counselor. In general, therapeutic services such as speech-language, occupational, and physical therapy are available to children with special health care needs that affect their education.

The professionals and families caring for children with cleft and craniofacial conditions need to work together to advocate for special education and therapy in the school system. Although a team approach is the preferred treatment paradigm for cleft-affected children, not all services can be provided conveniently in a cleft team setting in all instances. These treatments may sometimes need to be provided in the context of the patient's school environment (for example, therapy by the school's speech-language pathologist) with the help provided by education from specialists on the cleft team. Advocacy resources should be available to families through the offices of their local state legislators, education law centers, and university law schools and should be sought when barriers to cleft team outreach are encountered.

WHY IS CONTINUED ADVOCACY IMPORTANT?

Children with special health care needs are evaluated and treated in an interdisciplinary fashion, because consumers and practitioners alike have placed appropriate pressure on programs that support their care. It is now rare, for example, for a third-party payer to refuse payment for the repair of a cleft lip because it is considered cosmetic. This change occurred only because of the pressure brought by education and advocacy from both the consumers of treatment and the providers of treatment. Every time care providers mentor a student or appeal an insurance claim, they are essentially advocating for care. If the current level of care is to persist and evolve, those working in cleft-craniofacial services, whether in a laboratory or a hospital, need to continue to be vigilant and not complacent. Advocacy involves educating younger generations of practitioners, the general public, and legislators.

To ensure that care and advancements in diagnosis and treatment are available to patients with cleft and craniofacial conditions, major effort is needed by care providers and those engaging in related clinical and translational research. Every time a provider of care challenges a negative decision on the part of a third-party payer regarding a recommended treatment, that provider is advocating for the needs of affected individuals. Knowledge of every avenue that can be taken to change a negative decision regarding a recommended treatment or therapy further ensures that state-of-the-art care will be available to patients. Comments from consumers, providers, and researchers about legislative issues related to health care can help to maintain and increase the availability of interdisciplinary care. Many road blocks to care and research can be lifted through the education of legislators, government officials, and hospital and institutional officials, and this is probably one of the most effective forms of advocacy.

Advocacy efforts are enhanced by written data describing the beneficiaries of the effort, the nature of the intervention in question, and peer-reviewed data demonstrating the efficacy of the proposed program or project. Appeals against insurance denials, for example, should include all published data supporting the need for the procedure in question and the consequence to the patient if the procedure is not accomplished. It is beneficial to highlight the financial impact on the insurer for additional treatment necessitated by failure to perform the present treatment. School issues should be addressed in a similar manner. The staff in the offices of local and federal legislators can be helpful with many aspects of health care administration, including handling denials of supplemental Social Security income or school-based therapy. The administrative staff in legislative offices is usually knowledgeable about the regulations and laws regarding health care insurance, related pending legislation, and avenues for working with Social Security offices, school systems, and subsidized health insurance and Medicaid.

CONCLUSION

Health care advocacy is multifaceted. The role of cleft and craniofacial care providers in this process is as diverse as the care itself. To ensure the availability of appropriate care, as recommended by the American Cleft Palate-Craniofacial Association Parameters of Care and the Team Standards, providers and patients must work cooperatively and continuously to advocate by educating the public, legislators, school systems, health care systems, third-party payers, and those writing the curricula for related professional training programs.

3

Adopting a Cleft-Affected Child

Christin R. Lawrence

KEY POINTS

○ Adoptive parents of cleft-affected children share many similar experiences, and the journey comes with both joys and challenges.

○ Families should seek advice from a trusted medical professional and a licensed social worker before adopting a cleft-affected child. They may also choose to join social groups for added support.

○ Adoptive parents should connect with their local hospital, consult the craniofacial or cleft team before the child's arrival home, and write down their questions before attending surgical consultations.

○ The adoptive family's health insurance will automatically cover the internationally adopted child after arrival to the United States, but the family will be responsible for insurance deductibles and copays. Some states and countries help parents with some of the medical bills of a special-needs child.

This chapter is written for a specific audience—the adoptive parents of a cleft-affected child or prospective parents considering the adoption of a cleft-affected child. It discusses the experiences that the adoptive family of a child with *cleft lip* and/or palate may encounter. The chapter is not an exhaustive wealth of information, because it cannot capture the unique circumstances and specific needs of each family. However, many families have similar experiences that can encourage others when shared. This communication ensures adoptive families with a cleft-affected child that they are not alone in their journey.

SEEKING SUPPORT AND MEDICAL ADVICE BEFORE ADOPTION AND SURGERY

There are many reasons to build a family through adoption. Some people are naturally inclined to adopt and love a child who needs a home. Others choose to adopt because they are not able to have a child of their own. Some families choose domestic adoption, whereas others decide on international adoption. Regardless of the reason, the decision to adopt is a serious one that comes with particular responsibilities. Adopting a child with special needs—however correctable the special needs may be—presents additional challenges and hurdles. There are also a great many joys for all involved in bringing a child into a loving family. Preparation and education are essential to ensure that the adoptive child receives the care needed to thrive and grow to full potential. Not only will adoption dramatically change the life of the child, the adoptive family will also be forever changed.

It is advisable to seek guidance from a trusted medical professional and a licensed social worker before adopting a child with special medical needs. Such professionals can help to prepare the family for the medical, emotional, and financial realities of adopting a child with a cleft-related condition. They can also provide additional resources that the family can access for assistance and support throughout the child's life.

PERCEPTIONS AND REACTIONS FROM FAMILY, FRIENDS, AND STRANGERS

Cleft-affected children and their adoptive parents might be perceived differently by family, friends, and strangers. Cleft lip is a visible condition. Someone who has never been in contact with a person with a cleft can have many questions or certain reactions after seeing a cleft-affected child for the first time. Often, other children and sometimes adults will stare or ask blunt questions that are offensive or hurtful to the cleft-affected child and parent. Such behavior is particularly characteristic of children, who do not always intend to offend, but who simply react out of innocent curiosity.

It is natural for adoptive parents to want to react quickly and to protect their child from insensitive comments or the stares of others. A positive response would be to help their child know how to properly respond to such reactions or questions. Building trust from the beginning and letting their child know that he or she is loved and precious can help parents keep the lines of communication open. Adopted children should know that they can talk to their parents about their feelings regarding anything, especially the harsh words or reactions of others. Parents should educate their child, as well as others, about the proper way to respond in these situations. Education is critical. Well-educated parents can best educate others and advocate for their child in a caring manner.

Not all reactions are negative. Sometimes parents and children find support in the most unexpected places. In a public place such as a grocery store, for example, a stranger might notice the child and explain kindly that they too were born with a cleft lip or cleft palate. The person may offer polite encouragement or wish the child well with surgery.

Joining adoption-related social groups or those that involve parents of children with cleft lip and/or palate are helpful and supportive. These groups provide parents with support from peers and the opportunity to exchange ideas and experiences. Their children can get to know others who have a similar family dynamic, and they have the opportunity to befriend peers with whom they have a special need in common. This kind of social support is invaluable for the parents and child alike.

DISCUSSING SURGERY WITH THE CLEFT CARE TEAM

Some adoptive children have had no corrective surgery before coming home. Before the adoptive child's arrival home, proactive parents will connect with the local hospital and consult with the local cleft care team to discuss the timeline of necessary surgical procedures. Surgical revision may be needed for operations performed in the child's birth country.

If the adoptive family lives in an area with several local hospitals and has access to various craniofacial teams, they can meet with several physicians from the area. Parents should research the credentials and experience of the surgeon who will perform the surgery. Ultimately, parents need to choose the doctor they are most comfortable with and the team that best fits their child's specific needs. The hospital should be easily accessible, because the parents will be taking their child to appointments before surgery and for follow-up appointments for weeks after surgery. The child will likely need to stay overnight in the hospital after the surgery, and occasionally only one parent will be allowed to stay in the room. These are only a few of the logistic factors to consider when choosing a surgical team/hospital.

Once a hospital and cleft care team are chosen, the long wait begins. This is the time to prepare as much as possible before the child comes home. It is an exciting time, but it can also be a time that causes anxiety for the family. These emotions are to be expected. It is good to spend the time and nervous energy preparing for the child's arrival and being proactive about future care in every way.

The adoptive family can request updates on their child's medical information from the adoption agency, foster parents, or the social welfare institute or orphanage. Often, especially with international adoptions, the information is not extensive, timely, or completely accurate. Nevertheless, adoptive parents should share with the physician all of the information they can obtain regarding their child's medical and developmental status. This information will be helpful for planning future care and surgical procedures, and it can help adoptive parents become more comfortable with potential obstacles and increase their understanding of the procedures their child will need in the future. Frequently, the physician does not know what is needed for a patient until the first in-person examination.

Families can ask their local hospital about adoptive support for families who have children with special medical needs. Some hospitals have a separate department or clinic for this purpose (for example, an international adoption clinic). Such a clinic of professionals can help the family understand how their child is progressing developmentally. Families can ask questions about caring for their child on arrival into their family.

An established relationship with such medical professionals is a beneficial resource for adoptive parents before they bring their child home. For example, if a family is adopting internationally, they might discover that their child is ill with a fever. They can contact the physician with whom they have a relationship and ask for help and advice.

After adoptive parents bring their child home and settle in, they should take their child to the first appointment with the primary care physician, international adoption clinic, or craniofacial team. This appointment will begin with a general examination of the child. The physician will most likely test the child's blood for needed immunizations. The physician or surgeon will assess the child's cleft and determine the surgical timeline. Providers may also evaluate the child for hearing loss and behavioral, developmental, dental, and speech issues.

FEEDING

Many parents investigate various methods of feeding their cleft-affected child and are surprised to find that the information is focused on caring for an infant. The child may have already learned how to eat in a different manner than the adoptive parents have prepared for, especially if the cleft lip and/or palate is not repaired before adoption. This is often the case for children adopted internationally (Fig. 3-1).

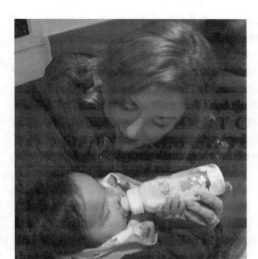

Fig. 3-1 Sophie's first feeding with her mother in China.

Special cleft bottles can be purchased online for children of bottle-feeding age. Particularly before international adoptions, it is helpful to purchase these bottles a couple of months in advance. They can be packed for the trip to pick up the child. The child may have already learned to eat from a regular, inexpensive bottle with a large slit cut in the nipple. It may seem as if the child is chugging the formula or milk. The child may have learned out of necessity how to eat from these bottles provided by the orphanage. This method of feeding can cause them to eat too fast or lead to difficulty with choking or digestion if the hole is cut too large.

Orphanages do the best they can with limited resources. It is a good gesture to take extra cleft bottles to gift to the orphanage or social welfare institute in the country. In some countries such as China, these special bottles are not readily available or are too expensive for families to obtain. Other cleft-affected children who are or will be in the orphanage's care will greatly benefit from bottles that help them to feed with the least possible amount of difficulty. For more information about feeding children with cleft-related conditions, see Chapter 7.

Many adopted children are able to eat soft solid foods by the time they arrive in their new homes. Adoptive parents need to be aware that food might come out of their child's nose because of the open palate. Such events can be difficult at first for parents. Parents become accustomed to the routine, and meals quickly become less messy by the time surgery to repair the palate takes place.

For children born with cleft lip and palate, lip repair is usually performed first. However, the parents and surgeon may decide to slightly delay the lip surgery after considering a range of issues, such as the child's overall health, age, development, trust, and emotional attachment. The formation of emotional attachment between adoptive parents and their child is vitally important in the beginning of an adoption. Doctors and parents do not want to disrupt this attachment by performing surgery too soon. As long as the child is able to eat and gain the weight necessary for proper growth and development, it is perfectly acceptable to delay the surgery (Fig. 3-2).

The timing of surgery for a newborn with cleft palate depends on the child's health, age, and the collective decision of the parents and craniofacial team. If the cleft child has a repaired cleft lip, the palate surgery will be scheduled to take place after

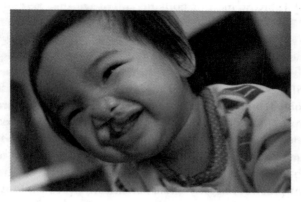

Fig. 3-2   Sophie before lip surgery.

the lip is fully healed. Depending on the child, palate surgery is usually performed at about 1 year of age. For adopted children with cleft lip and palate who come to their new home at an older age, surgery to repair the lip and palate might occur in the reverse order to more quickly provide an intact mechanism for speech production. In such cases, the palate may be repaired before the lip.

FUNDING AND INSURANCE

An adoptive family's health insurance will automatically cover an internationally adopted child after arrival to the United States; however, the parents will be responsible for paying the cost of the deductible and copays. The parents might need to travel to the hospital or clinic for preoperative care, surgery, and postoperative care. They may need to miss days from work. See Chapter 11 for information about how the craniofacial team social worker can help to manage these responsibilities.

Some states and countries have funds available to assist parents with medical bills for a child with special needs. The adoptive parents should contact the local authorities or their licensed social worker to obtain information about available resources.

CONCLUSION

Every child is special, and all children have the same basic needs such as a loving family, a safe home, food, water, clothes, and available medical care. A child who is adopted will need even more love, patience, and understanding.

After the immediate stress of surgery subsides, the child is stronger and able to thrive. The child can eat without difficulty and has improved speech and more confidence. The child, parents, and siblings can grow stronger as a family as they learn to trust and depend on one another through these experiences (Fig. 3-3).

Parents of children with cleft lip and palate often reminisce fondly about the early months and years after adopting their child. They look at pictures of their young baby or small child and compare them to later photos that show the child's progress. This reflection brings cherished memories of their child at the time of adoption and an abundance of gratitude for how far they have come as a family (Fig. 3-4).

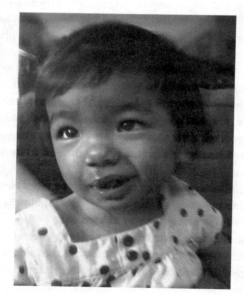

Fig. 3-3   Sophie 1½ weeks after cleft lip surgery.

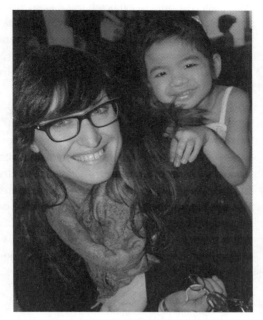

Fig. 3-4   Sophie and her mother at ballet class.

Classification of Orofacial Clefts

Mark P. Mooney

KEY POINTS

- The significant variability of orofacial clefts makes the creation of a single classification system difficult.

- The various needs of medical and rehabilitation professionals add to the difficulty of developing a single classification system.

- Some have attempted to create classification systems based on anatomy, developmental stage, and genetics.

- No one classification system addresses all these needs.

Orofacial clefts (OFCs) are caused by many factors and have many different forms. An accurate classification is needed for proper surgical and clinical management, genetic counseling, and research. Many classification systems for OFCs have been proposed and used over the years. These systems are based on detailed descriptions of the morphology (shape and anatomic structure), development, and genetic causes of OFCs. This chapter presents a short review of currently used OFC classification systems and discusses the common characteristics that make such classification systems useful (or not) to specific disciplines. Orofacial clefts are described as unilateral (Fig. 4-1) or bilateral (Fig. 4-2) clefts of the lip with or without a cleft of the palate (CL/P), isolated clefts of the palate (Fig. 4-3), or orofacial clefts (Fig. 4-4).

The Centers for Disease Control and Prevention (CDCP) studied birth differences and reported that OFCs are the most common birth difference in the United States, with a birth prevalence of 16.87/10,000 live births. The prevalence of OFCs varies by

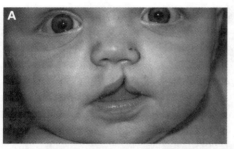

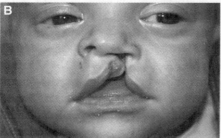

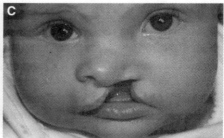

Fig. 4-1   Variability in unilateral orofacial clefts. **A,** An incomplete unilateral cleft lip. **B,** A narrow, complete unilateral cleft lip and cleft palate. **C,** A wide, complete unilateral cleft lip and cleft palate.

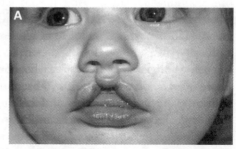

Fig. 4-2   Variability in bilateral orofacial clefts. **A,** An incomplete bilateral cleft lip. **B,** A complete and incomplete bilateral cleft lip and cleft palate. **C,** A complete bilateral cleft lip and cleft palate.

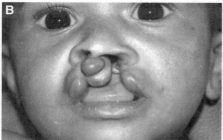

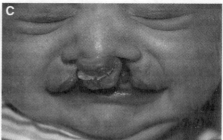

Fig. 4-3   Variability in palatal clefts. **A,** A *submucous cleft palate.* **B,** A *bifid uvula.* **C,** A complete unilateral cleft lip and cleft palate.

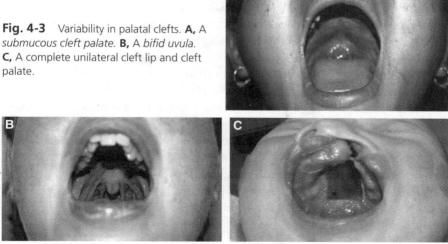

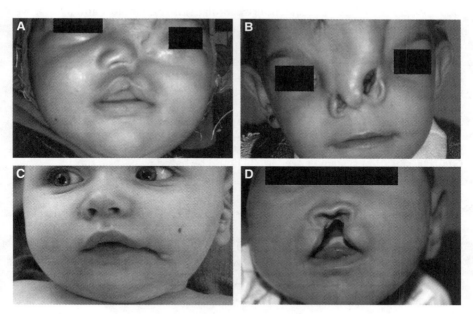

Fig. 4-4   Variability in rare orofacial clefts. **A,** A Tessier number 1 and number 14 orofacial cleft. **B,** A Tessier number 3 orofacial cleft. **C,** A Tessier number 7 orofacial cleft. **D,** A Tessier number 14 orofacial cleft. (See Morphologically Based Classification Systems for a discussion of the Tessier classification system.)

race, gender, and income. Native American and Asian populations have the highest birth prevalence for CL/P (15.0 to 36.0/10,000 live births), followed by European populations (10.0/10,000 live births). African populations have the lowest birth prevalence for CL/P (5.0/10,000 live births). Males are more likely than females to have CL/P, and females are more likely than males to have a cleft palate. For unilateral clefts, the ratio of left-sided/right-sided clefts is approximately 2:1. Babies born in rural areas with lower income levels have a higher risk for CL/P, compared with those from similar ethnic groups born in more urban areas with higher incomes.

The severity of OFCs varies tremendously and the causes are complex, which makes them difficult to classify. OFCs can occur as part of single gene mutations, chromosomal anomalies, or as the result of *prenatal* exposure to certain drugs and environmental factors. A lot of progress has been made in recent years in identifying gene disorders; this accounts for only a small number of people with orofacial clefts.

A child's cleft can be part of a group of congenital differences, or it can be the child's only difference. This information helps to determine the clinical and surgical management, to assess recurrence risk for patients and families, and to improve genetic analysis. Major birth differences are defined as those of functional or cosmetic significance needing some degree of medical intervention; minor differences are defined as those of minimal or no cosmetic or functional significance, which occur in less than 5% of the population.

The wide variety of types and sites of orofacial clefting—with or without associated birth anomalies in other parts of the body—has made the development of a single classification system of OFCs very difficult. A consistent and biologically accurate OFC classification system is needed. It should be based in part on our increasing knowledge of prenatal development and craniofacial genetics. In addition, with the recent identification and better understanding of the specific genes involved with orofacial clefting, both of these factors (differences in prenatal development and specific gene mutations) may be useful in developing a more accurate classification system of OFC. This classification would be partly based on specific genetic mutations and the timing of when the cleft occurs during craniofacial development, rather than solely on how a child looks at birth.

OROFACIAL CLEFT CLASSIFICATION SYSTEMS

An accurate classification of each patient is essential for appropriate surgical and clinical management, genetic counseling, and research. However, the many different scientific and medical specialists who need and use this information have not been able to agree on a universally acceptable and usable classification system.

Craniofacial surgeons need specific information regarding structural and anatomic problems for presurgical planning. Orthodontists, speech-language pathologists, psychologists, and genetic counselors draw conclusions about treatment outcomes and recurrence risk rates based on the cause of the cleft (if known) and not necessarily the appearance of the cleft.

The following sections present short reviews of currently used OFC classification systems based on morphology, development, and genetic causes, including the common characteristics that make such classification systems useful (or not) to specific disciplines.

Morphologically Based Classification Systems

Early OFC classifications coincided with the "modern" era of surgery after World War I. During this time, reconstructive surgeons began applying procedures for treating battlefield trauma for facial reconstruction in children born with OFCs.

In 1931 a surgeon named Victor Veau presented a widely accepted system for classifying oral clefts into four subgroups known as Veau cleft types. This system is still very popular (Fig. 4-5). Using this classification system, surgeons could communi-

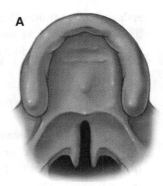

Fig. 4-5   Veau classification. **A,** Type I: Clefts of the soft palate only. **B,** Type II: Complete clefts of the soft and hard palate. **C,** Type III: Complete unilateral cleft of the hard and soft palate that usually includes a unilateral cleft lip. **D,** Type IV: Complete bilateral cleft of the hard and soft palate that usually includes a bilateral cleft lip.

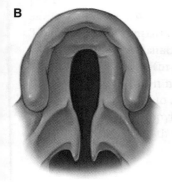
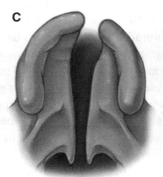
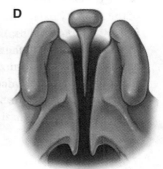

cate with one another about the anatomic nature of the cleft in their patients, and researchers could classify OFCs according to an operational definition for which classes were grouped together for clinical studies.

These early classification systems were based only on anatomy and were used sporadically by clinicians and researchers. They were designed by surgeons to specify particular cleft types for management and research, but they failed to gain much popularity with other researchers outside the surgical community. They are limited because they do not recognize many important factors such as the complex causes of OFC, which are critical in diagnosis and management. Some of the morphologically (shape and structure) based classification categories are overgeneralized.

Several studies have attempted to classify rare facial clefts according to anatomic and morphologic characteristics. In 1976 Paul Tessier proposed an anatomic and descriptive classification system in which unusual facial clefts are numbered based on their position relative to the eye socket, similar to spokes on a wheel, where the eye is at the center (see Figs. 4-4 and 4-6). Clefts are numbered from 0 (a midline cleft of the lip and nose) to 30 (a cleft of the *mandible*). The Tessier classification provides an anatomic description of the location and extent of facial clefts and is widely used by surgeons. However, it is not comprehensive, because it does not describe the extent and type of affected tissues or the cause of the OFCs. Thus this classification system is less useful to nonsurgical specialists such as orthodontists, speech-language pathologists, and genetic counselors.

Developmentally Based Classification Systems

As knowledge and understanding of developmental and craniofacial biology increased, classification systems based on early developmental events were created. Many of these systems attempted to correlate clinical features of OFCs with the timing of cleft events during early prenatal development.

Ross and Johnston developed one such system based on the knowledge that the palate develops in two parts: the primary palate and the secondary palate. Clefts of the primary palate involve the lip and the part of the *hard palate* in front of the *incisive foramen.* Clefts of the secondary palate involve the hard palate behind the incisive foramen and the *soft palate* (Fig. 4-7). Another classification system needs to be used for intensive genetic studies that require precise data and numerous subgroups related to laterality (right-sided or left-sided clefts) and cleft severity in each anatomic region.

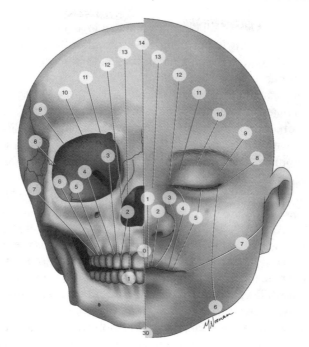

Fig. 4-6   Tessier orofacial cleft classification. Clefts are numbered from 0 (a midline cleft of the lip and nose) to 30 (a mandibular cleft).

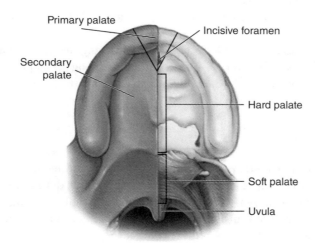

Fig. 4-7   The primary palate is the portion of the palate in front of the incisive foramen. The secondary palate is behind the incisive foramen. In the right side of the figure, the soft tissue covering of the palate (the mucosa) has been removed to show the structures underneath.

Classification systems based on development can give more information about the mechanisms producing OFCs, compared with morphologically based classification systems. However, developmentally based classification systems have the following limitations:

- They do not explain the cause of the OFC.
- They do not acknowledge the amount of individual variation of OFCs.
- They do not describe the range of other noncraniofacial medical conditions often seen with OFCs.
- They do not provide sufficient information regarding possible recurrence risks.

Genetically Based Classification Systems

Despite the many genetic causes of OFCs, most cleft patients are treated in the same way regardless of the cause. One reason is our inability to treat each patient in the most efficient manner according to the specific cause of the OFC. Some OFC conditions require different modes of management. Pharyngeal flaps, for example, are highly effective in treating the *velopharyngeal insufficiency* that often occurs after repair of a cleft palate (see Chapter 25). However, they may cause problems in patients with *Treacher Collins syndrome* because of the high potential for upper airway obstruction. As another example, primary repair of the palate in *22q11.2 deletion syndrome,* also known as *velocardiofacial syndrome,* may not result in a successful speech outcome. Thus, in theory, some clinical and surgical treatments can be tailored to the patient's OFC condition, based in part on the genetic classification and not exclusively on the morphologic or developmental classification.

Great strides have been made recently in identifying the genetic basis of OFCs. Classifications based on known genetic causes are being developed and combined with morphologically and developmentally based systems.

CONCLUSION

Many classification systems of OFCs have been proposed and used. These systems are based on detailed descriptions of the morphologic, developmental, and genetic causes of OFCs. However, most of these classification systems are discipline dependent and do not translate well across medical specialties. Practical applications of these classification systems show that they can be improved. In theory, a classification system that combines information on the morphology, development, and genetic cause of OFCs would be most useful, but such a unifying classification system has yet to be developed.

5

Prenatal Genetic Counseling

Donna M. McDonald-McGinn, Lauren DiCairano,
Kelsey Smith, Michael Mennuti

KEY POINTS

○ Prenatal detection of a cleft can help a family prepare psychologically and practically for the arrival of their child.

○ Prenatal detection allows families to form an early relationship with a cleft/craniofacial team.

○ Genetic counseling can provide important information about other conditions possibly associated with a child's cleft.

○ Genetic counselors can provide information about a cleft-affected patient's risk of having a child with a cleft.

○ Genetic counselors can be an important source of psychosocial support for cleft-affected patients and their families.

A prenatal diagnosis of a cleft lip and/or cleft palate can be devastating news to the family, regardless of the severity of the condition. Generally, the diagnosis comes as a surprise to families who are expecting to have a perfectly healthy baby. They might mourn the loss of the expected, normal child while learning new information about what this finding will mean to their child and the entire family. The attitude of the health care professional delivering the news, the diagnostic evaluations that will follow, and the opportunity to discuss the diagnosis with experienced professionals and support organizations can substantially reduce the burden on the family. In hindsight, many couples consider the prenatal diagnosis of a cleft lip and/or palate an important benefit, because it allows the family and medical staff to prepare for the birth of the affected child.

REFERRAL TO A GENETIC COUNSELOR

Typically, families meet with a *genetic counselor* because of a family history of a cleft lip and/or palate or after the child's cleft is diagnosed during routine prenatal ultrasonography. Once a cleft is diagnosed, additional questions arise regarding the cause, what to expect in the long term, potential treatment options, and the risk for future pregnancies. The genetic counselor can provide answers to many of the family's questions using a systematic diagnostic process to obtain an accurate diagnosis.

ESTABLISHING A PRENATAL CLEFT DIAGNOSIS

Prenatal detection of a cleft was first reported more than three decades ago. Facial clefts are usually diagnosed prenatally with an ultrasound evaluation. A cleft can be detected as early as the end of the first trimester of pregnancy. However, most are diagnosed during a routine ultrasound examination in the second trimester, from 18 to 22 weeks of pregnancy. If the family has a known history of cleft lip and/ or palate, detection can occur earlier. The detection rate varies greatly depending on numerous factors such as the experience of the ultrasound technician, the quality of the imaging equipment, and the position of the fetus during the scan. Examples of several available technologies include two-dimensional and three-dimensional ultrasound imaging and fetal magnetic resonance imaging (MRI). A two-dimensional evaluation of the baby mainly focuses on the nose, the lower jaw, the lip, and the palate. Supplemental three-dimensional ultrasound or fetal MRI might be recommended to confirm the presence or absence of a suspected cleft. In addition, three-dimensional images show the baby's features in more detail. However, ultrasound imaging is not capable of identifying a cleft lip and/or palate in every affected fetus.

Establishing a specific diagnosis, especially during pregnancy, is complex and requires multiple components. These often include a complete family history, laboratory testing, and possibly referrals to subspecialists to rule out a preexisting genetic condition in one of the parents.

The genetic counselor will ask the family about their health history for the last several generations, including relatives with clefts or other medical issues such as heart disease, eye problems, and hearing loss. The answers to these questions can be clues to conditions that run in the family. The genetic counselor often asks about previous birth defects, multiple miscarriages, learning disabilities, behavioral health issues in the family, and whether the mother took particular medications during pregnancy.

Once a cleft is identified or suspected, the follow-up ultrasound evaluation generally includes a scan for other birth defects. The presence of an additional finding can be a clue to an underlying condition or syndrome (a group of findings that tend to occur together), and further testing is often recommended. Frequent evaluations will monitor for growth disorders such as growth restriction and other differences that may be more easily visualized later in pregnancy. Fetal echocardiography, three-dimensional or four-dimensional ultrasonography, and fetal MRI are sometimes recommended as additional screening tests or to view other findings in more detail. The genetic counselor can provide answers to many of the family's questions about these tests and results.

Every cell in our body contains 23 pairs of chromosomes, which are the structures that carry genes. Genes are made of deoxyribonucleic acid (DNA), which is the genetic material or blueprint that determines traits such as eye color, hair color, and height. Typically, babies inherit one copy of each gene from their father and one copy of the same gene from their mother. Tests can be performed before the baby is born to look for differences in chromosomes or changes in genes that are sometimes associated with clefts. Examples of these tests include *chorionic villus sampling* and *amniocentesis*. Chorionic villus sampling is performed between 10 and 13 weeks of gestation and involves obtaining a sample from the placenta, which contains chromosomes from the fetus. Amniocentesis is generally performed at approximately 16 weeks of gestation and involves obtaining a sample of amniotic fluid (fluid surrounding the fetus), which contains fetal skin cells that can be analyzed for changes in the genes or chromosomes. It is usually offered to families if a cleft is suspected during the anatomy ultrasound evaluation, which is typically performed between 18 and 22 weeks of gestation. Additional, more sophisticated, laboratory studies can also be performed if needed. After tests are completed, families find it very beneficial to meet with specialists to discuss the findings and other potential implications for their baby's health. These specialists usually include a plastic surgeon, an otolaryngologist, and a geneticist. Depending on results of the prenatal tests, families might also meet with a cardiologist, a neurologist, a neurosurgeon, an orthopedic surgeon, and/or an ophthalmologist.

In addition to the results of genetic testing, the type of cleft can provide clues to the underlying cause and help to narrow the possible associated diagnoses. For instance, a midline cleft can be associated with a condition in the brain called holoprosencephaly, in which the front part of the brain does not develop properly. Developmental delays and seizures are common in these patients, some of whom do not survive beyond the first few days of life. Holoprosencephaly has many causes such as an extra or missing chromosome. (Too much or too little chromosome material can cause a problem in the development of the fetus.) One common cause is trisomy 13 (an extra chromosome 13). Holoprosencephaly can also be associated with a change in a single gene (a genetic mutation). Sometimes one of the parents has the same change and yet has no symptoms. This is called variable expressivity—the same mutation can have various effects in different people of the same family. Holoprosencephaly can occur if the fetus is exposed to a teratogen (a nongenetic cause). Examples of teratogens that can cause holoprosencephaly include uncontrolled diabetes in the mother and fetal exposure to alcohol or retinoic acid (a medication used to treat acne).

UNILATERAL OR BILATERAL CLEFT LIP AND/OR PALATE

A unilateral or bilateral cleft lip and/or palate is diagnosed in approximately 1 in 1000 newborn babies. These clefts can result from differences in chromosomes or genes, exposure to teratogens during fetal development, or sporadic conditions, in which no known genetic or environmental cause is identified.

Chromosomal differences most commonly associated with clefts include trisomies (in particular trisomy 13, as previously mentioned), Wolf-Hirschhorn syndrome (a deletion [absence] of genes on chromosome 4), 22q11.2 deletion syndrome (deletion of a small piece of chromosome 22), and many other deletions or duplications (an extra copy of a gene) that typically cause varying physical and intellectual differences. A genetic test called a chromosome microarray can detect deletions and/or duplications in the chromosomes and can be performed after a cleft is identified.

In contrast to chromosomal differences, changes in genes (mutations) have more variable effects on the body. Problems caused by single-gene changes are well described but relatively rare conditions. Examples include Van der Woude syndrome and popliteal pterygium syndrome. Both of these are caused by mutations in the gene known as IRF6. Both syndromes include cleft lip, cleft lip and palate, cleft palate only, absent teeth, and lip pits. In addition to these findings, popliteal pterygium syndrome also causes differences in the area behind the knees (the popliteal region). Other examples of single-gene changes that cause physical differences include Rapp-Hodgkin ectodermal dysplasia and ectrodactyly–ectodermal dysplasia cleft syndrome. Both syndromes are caused by a mutation in the gene known as P63. Both syndromes include a cleft lip or cleft lip and palate and varying problems with hair, teeth, and nails, but patients with ectrodactyly–ectodermal dysplasia cleft syndrome also have limb differences. These are autosomal dominant conditions, meaning a person only needs one affected copy of the involved gene for the condition to be present. These mutations can be inherited from either parent (familial) or they can occur randomly during early development (de novo).

On the other hand, autosomal recessive conditions require changes in both copies of a gene (the copy from the mother and the copy from the father). If a child has an autosomal recessive condition, both parents are usually carriers, meaning each has one working and one nonworking gene for the specific condition. Carriers are typically healthy and not affected by the nonworking gene. An example of an autosomal recessive condition associated with clefting is oral-facial-digital syndrome, type VI, which causes a cleft lip and palate and differences in the fingers and toes.

An example of a condition that is associated with clefting but is not hereditary is fetal hydantoin (Dilantin) syndrome. This can occur if a child's mother had to take Dilantin to control her seizures during the pregnancy.

All of these associations support additional prenatal imaging studies when a cleft is identified, as well as a thorough family/pregnancy history and parental examinations.

The cause of cleft palate is thought to be different from that of cleft lip. Cleft palate is often more difficult to detect on prenatal ultrasound evaluations, and it is more common, occurring in 1 of 2500 live births. It has multiple causes, including chromosomal abnormalities; autosomal dominant conditions such as Van der Woude syndrome and Stickler syndrome; autosomal recessive conditions such as Smith-Lemli-Opitz syndrome; exposure to teratogens such as alcohol or Dilantin; and generally sporadic conditions with unknown causes.

PIERRE ROBIN SEQUENCE

Pierre Robin sequence is a well-recognized condition characterized by micrognathia (a smaller than normal jaw) and glossoptosis (the tongue falls back and obstructs the airway); it can occur with or without a cleft palate. The exact cause is unknown but is thought to be a combination of genetic and environmental factors. Some associated chromosomal causes include deletions of genes 4q, 6q, and 22q11.2 and duplications of 11q. Examples of associated single-gene disorders include Stickler syndrome and Treacher Collins syndrome. Pierre Robin sequence can result from exposure to teratogens, including alcohol, Dilantin, and trimethadione (another antiseizure medication). Another environmental cause of cleft palate is oligohydramnios (the presence of less amniotic fluid than normal in the womb), which restricts fetal movements in the womb.

Isolated occurrences of Pierre Robin sequence are common. Therefore, if it is suspected in an unborn baby, for example, one with holoprosencephaly, numerous causes are possible. Stickler syndrome and 22q11.2 deletion syndrome are the most common genetic causes. Additional imaging and laboratory studies can help to eliminate some of the possible causes. Babies with Pierre Robin sequence can have breathing difficulties; careful planning by a multidisciplinary health care team is required to prevent complications during and after delivery.

ISOLATED CLEFTS

Most clefts occur as an isolated finding (not in addition to one of the previously described syndromes) or in combination with other physical differences not associated with a known condition. Therefore, parents are relieved to learn that their child might not have additional medical problems. Furthermore, a cleft lip and palate appears to have different implications than a cleft palate alone. A relative of an individual with only a cleft palate has no greater chance of having a child affected with a cleft lip and palate than someone from the general population. Exceptions to this rule are cases in which cleft palate occurs as a part of a genetic diagnosis, such as in the 22q11.2 deletion or Van der Woude syndrome. In these disorders, cleft lip and/or palate and cleft palate alone may be observed within the same family. Therefore, these diagnoses should be considered when a family history includes both types of clefting.

MULTIFACTORIAL INHERITANCE AND RECURRENCE RISKS

An isolated cleft lip and/or palate is thought to have multifactorial inheritance (sporadic occurrence). This means that combinations of risk genes on both sides of the family are passed on to the child to increase the chance of developing a cleft. However, a nongenetic or environmental factor is also needed to push the baseline risk over a certain threshold, leading to the development of a cleft. The genetic cause has been well documented. In a family history with autosomal recessive inheritance (single-gene disorders), only one generation might have a cleft (for example, a child but not a parent or other relative). This lack of frequency is understandable. Because the condition requires two nonworking genes, one from each carrier parent, the recurrence risk is only 25%. In contrast, in a family with autosomal dominant inheritance (single-gene disorders), usually multiple generations have a cleft (for example, a parent and the child). Because the affected parent passes on his or her nonworking gene to the child, the recurrence risk is 50%.

The recurrence risks with multifactorial disorders, however, are much smaller than with single-gene disorders and can be influenced by the sex of the person with the cleft (male or female), the ethnic background (white, Asian, or black), and the severity of the condition (unilateral or bilateral). However, when three or more members of a nuclear family (which consists of the mother, the father, and their children) have a cleft, a single-gene disorder such as Van der Woude syndrome is usually suspected, even in the absence of other medical findings.

Nongenetic factors play a role in the severity of clefting. Although identical twins share the same genes, their clinical findings can be different—one may have a cleft, whereas the other does not. Likewise, a person's ethnic background can influence the risk of having a cleft lip and/or cleft palate. Asians have the highest risk at 14 in 10,000 births. The risk in whites and blacks is 10 in 10,000 and 4 in 10,000 births, respectively. Thus the recurrence risk for future children depends on many factors, including the sex of the affected person, the severity of the cleft, the ethnic background, and the number of affected family members.

When considering recurrence risks for cleft-affected individuals and their relatives, genetic counselors will distinguish multifactorial or sporadic clefting from clefting associated with chromosomal differences, single-gene disorders, teratogens, and isolated associations. For example, a unilateral cleft lip and palate is most often isolated, but can also occur in association with any of the following conditions: trisomy 13, Wolf-Hirschhorn syndrome, and fetal alcohol syndrome from maternal alcohol exposure. Genetic counseling for clefting must include a physical examination of all affected people and a thorough review of their medical records. Once a diagnosis has been made regarding the cause of the cleft, a genetic counselor can provide appropriate recurrence risk counseling and possible prenatal testing options.

PRECONCEPTION AND PRENATAL COUNSELING

Parents who have a family history of isolated clefting can benefit from meeting with a genetic counselor before conception. These meetings will include a discussion of folic acid supplementation. Numerous studies have shown that folic acid taken before conception reduces the occurrence and recurrence risk of clefting. Screening and diagnostic tests will be discussed, including various imaging options available during pregnancy.

For clefts associated with a family history of a genetic syndrome, prenatal options in addition to ultrasonography include fetal echocardiography, if congenital heart disease is associated with the condition, amniocentesis, and chorionic villus sampling. The discussion might include artificial insemination with sperm or a donor egg or a preimplantation genetic diagnosis with in vitro fertilization. Preimplantation genetic diagnosis is a screening test to detect a mutation or mutations in a single cell of an embryo before it is transferred to the uterus. In the future, new testing technologies such as noninvasive prenatal testing will be used early in pregnancy to screen for certain conditions associated with clefting. This will be a valuable option for families who wish to conceive without assistive technology such as in vitro fertilization.

The prenatal diagnosis of a cleft can have several advantages for families. It provides time to adjust to the unexpected news. The families' health care providers have time to consider possible underlying causes and pursue confirmatory testing. In some situations, a prenatal diagnosis provides time for the family and health care team to consider alternative plans for delivery, such as delivery in a larger facility than a community hospital. In addition, the family can meet with the cleft palate and/or craniofacial team to learn more about the potential surgical, speech, and feeding needs of their child, as well as the available resources for support and education in their area. This is the beginning of a long-term relationship that will ultimately contribute to the well-being of their child.

Despite the numerous advantages of a prenatal diagnosis, it can also negatively affect the family. If a family has not had the opportunity to bond with their baby, they can become anxious about the diagnosis of a cleft and the potential associated problems. This anxiety may lead to concerns about the prognosis and overall care and raise questions that may not be completely answered until after the birth of the child. In addition, many families feel guilt and blame themselves when told that their child has a birth defect. A genetic counselor can discuss the diagnosis, the prognosis, and the psychosocial concerns of the family. Some families will benefit from additional support. The genetic counselor can refer family members to an experienced mental health care provider, such as a psychologist, social worker (see Chapter 11), psychiatrist, or outside support groups.

POSTNATAL COUNSELING

Cleft-affected children and their siblings should receive genetic counseling as they enter adulthood. Counseling provides information about the recurrence risk for their children and provides psychosocial support. Although many children and adults with cleft lip and/or palate are not significantly affected psychosocially, some are teased about their scars (see Chapter 9). For some children, this presents difficult challenges. Caregivers should anticipate these concerns, support the patients and their families, and provide opportunities to ask for support.

CONCLUSION

Prenatal detection of a cleft lip and/or palate can help the family to prepare for the arrival of their child. Genetic counseling offers valuable information about other conditions possibly associated with the child's cleft. When families are introduced to their multidisciplinary cleft team before their baby's arrival, they can begin to establish relationships that will benefit the entire family through growth and development. As a cleft-affected child matures, genetic counselors can provide additional information about the risk of passing on the cleft trait to the next generation.

6

Prenatal Diagnosis and Consultation

Matthew D. Ford

KEY POINTS

○ Most orofacial clefts are identified in the second trimester of pregnancy. Prenatal diagnosis of infants with cleft lip is common because of ever-improving ultrasound technology and standardized testing; however, the technology has limitations.

○ Because of the limitations of ultrasound imaging, physicians are not always able to determine the severity of a cleft lip and whether the palate has a cleft. The inside of the mouth is difficult to view clearly. The unborn child's movements can also limit the effectiveness of the evaluation.

○ After the parents are informed of the diagnosis, they should be able to obtain a prenatal consultation with a cleft-craniofacial treatment center in a reasonable amount of time to help prepare for the birth of their child.

○ At the prenatal consultation, helpful information is discussed regarding necessary surgeries, medical insurance, feeding assistance, and the selection of a multidisciplinary cleft or craniofacial team, including the importance of the team's accreditation by the American Cleft Palate-Craniofacial Association (ACPA).

Because of advances in medical technology, the diagnosis of a cleft lip with or without a cleft palate is often made before the baby is born. Standard obstetric care typically involves an anatomic evaluation of the unborn child in the second trimester of pregnancy. This is the period when most orofacial clefts are identified. The diagnosis of a cleft can have an immediate impact on the mother and the entire family. Parents may feel grief, stress, and even fear, because answers to their many answers are unknown. A prenatal consultation with a cleft palate or craniofacial team can be useful in providing information to guide the family through this difficult time. Information that the parents receive at the consultation will help them develop realistic expectations.

PRENATAL DIAGNOSIS

A cleft lip and palate (orofacial clefting) is the most common birth defect in the United States, according to a report in 2006 from the Centers for Disease Control. One in every 598 children is born with an orofacial cleft. Because this diagnosis is so common, medical specialists have become increasingly knowledgeable in the diagnosis and management of cleft-related conditions. This leads to excellent treatment outcomes and patient satisfaction.

Ultrasound imaging is a part of routine obstetric care. Anatomic surveys are now a standard practice during prenatal care. In the second trimester of pregnancy, a level II ultrasound is typically performed. This evaluation is different from a regular ultrasound in that it provides more detailed, comprehensive information about the unborn child. Many body parts and organs are evaluated, including the heart, the limbs, the spine, the kidneys, the brain, the stomach, the genitalia, and the face. This test helps to identify many congenital differences that are possible. Cleft lip is one condition that is routinely identified.

Limitations in Prenatal Diagnosis of Cleft Lip or Palate

Ultrasound imaging is not a perfect science. Although it is a safe and noninvasive technology with a high degree of accuracy in diagnosing the presence of a cleft lip, it cannot be used for determining the severity of the cleft and whether the unborn child has a cleft palate. It can be a challenge to determine whether the cleft is complete (involving the lip, nose, and palate) or incomplete (affecting only a portion of the lip). Ultrasound imaging uses sound waves, which are mapped to form a picture of the baby's facial structures. With this technology, it is exceedingly difficult to look inside the mouth to confirm the presence of a cleft palate. The imaging is also limited by the baby's movements. The pictures can be obscured by a hand in the mouth, an arm across the face, or positioning within the womb. This is important information for parents to understand so that they can develop realistic expectations. In approximately 80% of infants diagnosed with a cleft lip, the palate is also involved to some degree.

Common Reactions From Parents

When an unborn child is diagnosed with an orofacial cleft, the parents often immediately want to know what they did wrong. They feel guilty, thinking that they may have done something to cause the cleft; most of the time this guilt is unfounded. On receiving the diagnosis, many parents will also feel grief, because they no longer have a perfect baby. This can place significant stress on the family. The excitement of pregnancy and having a newborn can be clouded by worrying about unanswered questions. The prenatal consultation should help the family answer some of these questions and better understand the diagnosis. The diagnosis of a cleft lip and/or palate does not prevent the child from becoming a healthy, productive adult. Most people who were born with a cleft condition lead productive lives and work in a variety of occupations. They have become movie actors, football players, politicians, and physicians. With proper treatment, these children will grow up to be healthy and happy, with friendships, families, and careers.

PRENATAL CONSULTATION

What to Expect After the Diagnosis

The parents are referred to a cleft treatment center after they receive the diagnosis. Usually, the mother's obstetrician will make this referral. Some families seek a treatment center on their own. Depending on the family's geographic location, the facility can be far away. For some families, multiple centers are close to home. The process of choosing a treatment center and a surgeon can be daunting. Families should contact the centers to ask about their treatment protocols (routine ways of treating the cleft). These vary between teams and centers. Most reputable institutions have fairly standardized treatment protocols. Parents should be able to obtain a prenatal consultation at a cleft-craniofacial treatment center in a reasonable amount of time to assist in preparing for their child's birth.

Prenatal consultations are commonly performed in most treatment centers. Any member of the team can provide the consultation. Frequently, it is conducted by one of the reconstructive surgeons, the pediatrician, or the team coordinator. (See Chapter 1 for a more complete discussion about the members of the cleft palate and craniofacial teams.) During the consultation, the family should feel comfortable requesting to see photographs of other children who have had similar clefts repaired. The following topics should be discussed during a prenatal consultation:

- The timing of the surgical repairs
- The use or availability of presurgical treatments to prepare a baby for surgery, such as taping, *nasoalveolar molding*, lip adhesion surgery, and others
- The availability of on-site multidisciplinary team members
- A complete list of on-site surgical interventions or where they are performed if they are not performed at the institution where the consultation takes place
- Type of medical insurance accepted
- The availability of outcome measures for quality assurance
- ACPA accreditation of the facility
- State/local programs that assist in payment for medical and surgical fees or access to care
- Feeding assistance for the newborn, including the availability of specialty feeding bottles and a cleft feeding specialist
- Instructions for initiating team care after the birth of the child

Parents should be able to easily obtain this information from a quality treatment team. The ACPA is a governing body that regulates minimum standards for team composition and quality of care. If a cleft palate or craniofacial team is not accredited by the ACPA, it is important to know why before an institution is selected.

A quality prenatal consultation should be comforting to the family. All of their questions should be answered. A contact person for the treatment team is designated; this is typically the team coordinator. The family should be able to easily obtain information from this person before and after delivery. The consultant outlines the team's philosophy of treatment and provides a general timeline of intervention, based on what is known about the diagnosis. The function of each team member is reviewed. The consultant will explain potential presurgical treatments and whether they are performed by the team and necessary for their child. If they are not offered, the consultant can explain why. Additionally, the consultant will discuss the family's eligibility for special programs that can help to pay for medical procedures, rehabilitation services, and access to additional services. This can ease the parents' concerns regarding the ability to pay for their child's care and the ability to access services if the clinic is far away.

Feeding the newborn is a critical part of the prenatal consultation (see Chapter 7). Infants born with a cleft involving the palate will have feeding challenges. Most infants are not delivered in the same medical center where they will receive cleft and/or craniofacial treatment. Many small community hospitals do not have access to specialty feeding bottles, and they do not employ experienced practitioners to assist in feeding an infant with a cleft palate. Parents should obtain contact information for one of the team's feeding specialists, who can provide support after the baby's birth.

The cleft palate and/or craniofacial team should explain why feeding can be challenging and show the family how to feed an infant with a cleft palate. The mother should have appropriate expectations about breast-feeding, because infants with cleft palate usually are not able to feed adequately from the breast. The feeding specialist will demonstrate appropriate feeding techniques and provide written resources. This information can reduce stress significantly.

INITIAL VISIT WITH THE TREATMENT TEAM

After the child is born, the parents should contact the treatment center to schedule the first visit. This should take place within the first few weeks of the delivery. At this visit, the infant's cleft will be diagnosed more precisely, and a comprehensive treatment plan will then be established. The family can participate in comprehensive team evaluations and begin the journey of multidisciplinary care that will lead to successful treatment.

CONCLUSION

Receiving the news that their unborn child has a cleft lip or other craniofacial difference can be devastating for parents. The information and care that a multidisciplinary cleft palate or craniofacial team can provide is essential. These teams are available in most parts of the United States and in many other countries. They consist of specialists from multiple disciplines who provide comprehensive treatment for children with cleft lip and/or palate. Access to a team is important for parents to obtain accurate information about needed treatment and to develop realistic long-term expectations. The ACPA provides accreditation to ensure that teams meet minimal standards for quality multidisciplinary care. Parents should begin to contact teams as soon as their child is diagnosed.

7

Nursing and Perioperative Care of the Child With Cleft Lip and Palate

Patricia D. Chibbaro, Mary Breen

KEY POINTS

o The responsibilities of the cleft lip and palate nurse specialist span the entire treatment experience of the child and family. This nurse is the important link between the family and the medical and surgical teams, providing ongoing education and support.

o The nurse specialist performs the key roles of coordinator of care and educator.

o Feeding the cleft-affected infant may be challenging and sometimes stressful for the family and the nursing staff. The nurse specialist educates caregivers about the types of available specialty feeding systems and works closely with them on the techniques needed for successful feeding.

o The nurse specialist plays an essential role in working with the nursing staff and the parents to provide safe and effective care for infants with Pierre Robin sequence. The specific areas of concern are maintenance of healthy breathing patterns and appropriate and safe feeding techniques.

The family of an infant with a cleft has many opportunities to interact with professional nurses. This relationship often begins during a prenatal consultation in which the family meets the nurse specialist on the cleft lip and palate team. Nurses work in the obstetric office, the hospital delivery room, the postpartum unit, the newborn nursery, and the neonatal intensive care unit. After the child is discharged, nurses and nurse practitioners will continue to provide care in the pediatric outpatient clinic or private pediatric office. When surgical procedures are scheduled, nurses in the operating and recovery rooms and the inpatient pediatric unit will deliver specialized surgical and postoperative care. The nurse specialist on the cleft lip and palate team is available as a consistent resource to the parents and family to help them understand and prepare for all phases of the child's treatment, including reconstructive surgeries. The roles and responsibilities of the cleft lip and palate nurse specialist may include the following:

- Cleft team member
- Patient care coordinator
- Prenatal nursing counselor
- Consultant to the birth hospital personnel
- Feeding instructor for the parents, birth hospital nursing staff, and other caregivers
- Comprehensive case manager for the patient and family
- Liaison for the patient, family, hospital staff, and community
- Preoperative and postoperative teaching
- Preoperative history-taking and physical assessment
- Education and support throughout nasoalveolar molding (NAM) therapy
- Postoperative inpatient and outpatient management
- Resource and in-service educator to pediatric nurses and house staff
- Community outreach and education

PRENATAL NURSING CONSULTATION

As a result of the advancements in ultrasound imaging, a prenatal cleft can be diagnosed as early as 18 weeks of gestation. Once the parents have been referred to a cleft treatment team, the cleft team nurse specialist is often the initial contact person. Some parents make contact within a few hours of receiving their child's diagnosis and are understandably emotional, distraught, and in a state of crisis. The cleft team members are there to help.

Many parent reports suggest that prior information gives the family an opportunity to research clefts and to identify a treatment team before the birth of the baby. Most agree that better preparation results in a more positive delivery and newborn experience. However, many couples relate that the rest of the pregnancy is more difficult because of the increased worry about the baby, including uncertainty about the severity of the cleft and other potential medical problems.

Protocols for prenatal consultation vary among teams. The visit may involve meetings with one or several members of the cleft team. Each has specific areas of expertise, but the information that they provide often overlaps. As information is presented, parents may become emotional and confused, often remembering little of what has been said. The nurse can be instrumental in helping parents deal with the news of the cleft by providing reassurance and accurate, nonjudgmental information.

Prenatal Nursing Consultation Timeline

During the prenatal nursing consultation, the parents and the nurse will share essential information. Throughout this process, the nurse has numerous responsibilities, including the following:
- The pregnancy history, delivery plans, and information about the family structure and resources are obtained.
- Information from prenatal meetings with the genetics counselor, the surgeon, and other cleft team members is clarified.
- Information that the parents have read on the Internet is explained.
- The parents' thoughts and feelings about the diagnosis are discussed and supported.
- The parents are assisted in expressing their concerns and verbalizing their fears. Parents usually want to know whether their baby will have other medical problems, how they will feed their baby, and whether the child will be able to have a normal life.
- Preoperative and postoperative medical photographs are reviewed.
- Feeding options are discussed and demonstrated, and samples of bottles and ordering information are provided.
- Advice is offered about how to explain the diagnosis to other family members and friends.
- A network with other parents of cleft-affected babies is provided.
- Nursing guidance is offered in preparation for preoperative NAM therapy.
- A brief explanation is provided for the expected hospital and postoperative care after the initial cleft lip and palate surgeries.

- The parents are referred to the Cleft Palate Foundation and Cleftline (1-800-24-CLEFT) and the website *(www.cleftline.org).*
- The parents are given cleft team literature and website information.
- The cleft team contact information is provided for the family and the hospital staff to call after the birth.

PREPARING FOR THE BIRTH OF THE BABY

The birth of the baby should be one of the family's happiest memories. One advantage of knowing the cleft diagnosis prenatally is that it provides the opportunity to ensure a positive birth experience. Parents should feel free to contact the labor and delivery and nursery staff before the delivery to inform them that their baby will be born with a cleft. They can also ask their obstetrician or pediatrician for help preparing the medical team.

Parents who receive a prenatal cleft diagnosis might be very anxious during the labor process. They may have been told that the baby could have additional medical problems, possibly a *syndrome.* Parents should know that the complete diagnosis, including the exact extent of the cleft lip and palate, can only be determined after their baby is delivered and evaluated by the medical team. The labor room nurse can provide tremendous emotional support, sensitivity about the parents' fears, and reassurance that the entire staff is prepared to assist in caring for the baby. This nurse can also be a liaison to the delivery room staff, alerting them in advance about the baby's cleft diagnosis and other medical problems that can be associated with the cleft.

If no emergent medical concerns arise, the infant should be treated as a typical newborn and does not need to automatically be placed in a neonatal intensive care unit (NICU). Some hospitals choose to monitor these babies in the NICU, because many of the nurses with expertise in specialized feeding techniques are assigned to this type of unit.

The medical team will examine the baby. Once the child is found to be otherwise healthy, the staff will explain the extent of the cleft to the parents. Sometimes immediate medical problems are noted at the time of the delivery, for example, in premature infants and those with a cardiac anomaly or Pierre Robin sequence. In this case, the parents will see their infant and are informed of the diagnosis before the baby is transferred to the NICU. They will be reunited with their baby in the NICU as quickly as possible. Often, because the mother needs more time to rest and recover from the birth, the father will be the first to see the baby. The nurses in the NICU are very sensitive to this situation and can provide additional emotional support as needed.

If the baby is placed in the NICU only for feeding support, the parents and nurses should advocate for the baby by minimizing "overtreatment." Babies with any type of palatal cleft can usually tolerate oral (by mouth) feedings. The immediate use of an orogastric, nasogastric, or gastrostomy tube for feeding (before an adequate trial of oral feeding with cleft palate feeders) is an example of overtreatment. This type of intervention may actually cause the infant to become very orally defensive, making bottle-feeding very difficult, even with the proper equipment and feeding techniques. It is acceptable to question the medical team about the reasons for specific aspects of the baby's treatment. Parents who have already met with a cleft team should share their team's contact information with the doctors and nurses. Parents should ask them to consult with the cleft team for advice.

An otherwise healthy infant with a cleft can be transferred directly from the delivery room to the newborn nursery. The nurses caring for the baby can be instructed on feeding methods, either by NICU nurses with experience feeding children with a cleft, a feeding specialist, the cleft palate nurse clinician at the hospital, or the nurse on the cleft team with whom the parents met prenatally. Parents can contact the Cleft Palate Foundation's Cleftline for additional support. They will then be referred to a cleft team specialist who can assist with feeding by phone. Parents who received feeding instruction and/or supplies during the prenatal consultation may need to teach the newborn nursing staff how to feed the baby.

DISCHARGE FROM THE HOSPITAL

Ideally, the baby and mother are discharged together from the hospital if the child has no other medical concerns and is starting to take enough feedings by mouth (see Feeding the Cleft-Affected Infant in this chapter). The following checklist can be helpful for parents before they leave the hospital:
- The baby's type of cleft was explained.
- Instructions for feeding techniques were provided (and we are starting to feel comfortable using them).
- Feeding supplies were provided (for parents who do not have them at home).
- A referral to a lactation consultant was provided (for mothers who plan to breast-feed).
- A record of the baby's birth and discharge weights was provided.
- The goals for feeding (number of ounces per day if bottle-feeding) were explained.

- We met with or were given a referral to a social worker in case we need assistance, for example, dealing with our feelings about the baby and managing reactions of siblings, other family members, and the public.
- Appointments have been made with the cleft team and primary care provider (pediatrician or nurse practitioner).
- Information was provided for locating a team through the Cleft Palate Foundation (for parents who have not already contacted a team).

NURSING CARE OF AN INFANT UNDERGOING NASOALVEOLAR MOLDING THERAPY

Some cleft teams offer presurgical NAM therapy, also known as PNAM. This involves placement of a removable acrylic appliance that serves to bring the lip, gum, and nose into better alignment. The surgeon and/or orthodontic team will explain NAM therapy to the parents either during the prenatal consultation or the first team visit after the child is born. The cleft team nurse will then review and clarify the information with the parents. Parents will be given literature about the treatment and the contact information for other families who are willing to share their experience with NAM therapy. This networking is optional, but it can help to answer questions best addressed by other parents whose children have undergone this therapy.

Before the child begins NAM therapy, the parents will meet with the orthodontic team to discuss the management of weekly or biweekly appointments, travel, associated financial concerns, and additional maternity or family medical leave that may be needed. NAM therapy can be a challenging but very manageable, positive team effort. The parents share equal importance with the surgeon and the dental and orthodontic team in the baby's care and in the outcome of the surgery.

During the initial visit, the nurse will discuss some potential NAM-related feeding issues. Many parents think that they will be able to successfully breast-feed their infant with the NAM appliance in place, especially if the cleft involves only the lip, nose, and alveolus (gum) and if the infant was able to latch on and feed adequately after birth. If the child has a cleft palate, parents often assume that the NAM appliance will cover the palatal opening and that the baby can then successfully breast-feed. However, experience at most centers has shown that the baby will not be able to breast-feed once the NAM appliance has been inserted (ideally by 2 to 3 weeks of age), because often the experience is not comfortable for the mother or the infant. Removing the appliance for nursing is discouraged; it can actually separate the alveolar (gum) segments, essentially undoing the work that has been accomplished. Many parents report, however, that after the NAM appliance has been inserted and the baby has a few days to adjust to it, feeding seems to improve. Feeding will probably improve with time, the use of the proper bottles, and experience with various techniques, because most babies with a cleft of the palate only (who are not fitted with a molding appliance or obturator/feeding plate), improve with feeding on their own within the first month of life.

Once the parents are ready to proceed with NAM therapy, the dentist or orthodontist will make an impression of the infant's alveolus to custom-make the molding appliance. The dental hygienist can describe the procedure and ensure that it will be completed in a few moments. The dental hygienist will also reassure the parents that their baby will be safe and carefully monitored by the dental or orthodontic team. While the impression is made, the nurse specialist can stay with the parents. This is a good time for the parents to ask questions about feeding and the treatment plan and to express any concerns about adjusting to having a new baby. The team social worker can also meet with the parents at this visit (see Chapter 11). The NAM appliance is then made. This may take several days, depending on whether it is made on-site or sent to an outside laboratory.

Once the NAM appliance is ready for use, the parents and the baby will return to the dental or orthodontic team's office for the appliance insertion. Many teams will demonstrate the insertion and taping process using a doll, because this is a much less stressful way for parents to learn (Fig. 7-1). When the parents are comfortable with the technique, the baby's appliance can be inserted. The baby may need a few days to adjust to the appliance. During this time, feeding and sleeping might be affected.

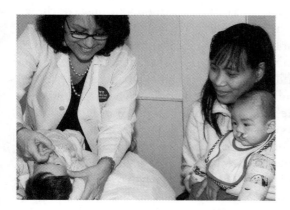

Fig. 7-1 The orthodontic team administrator uses a doll to demonstrate the proper taping of the NAM appliance.

Protocols for the care and management of the molding appliance will differ between cleft centers. Parents should receive clear, written instructions. In general, the appliance is removed daily for cleaning. The use of a soft toothbrush with warm water and a small amount of toothpaste is recommended. The appliance should not be boiled. Parents will be instructed to periodically place a finger in the baby's mouth while the appliance is in place to examine it for any sharp edges that might irritate the tongue. A penlight and cotton swab can be used to examine the gums for areas of irritation.

The appliance is generally secured in the mouth with a taping process. Base tapes are first placed on the cheeks to help prevent skin irritation from the frequent removal and replacement of the retention tapes that are attached to the appliance. Examples of base tapes include Tegaderm, Duoderm, and hydrocolloid bandages. The base tape needs to remain dry to prevent skin breakdown. The tapes remain in place for up to 3 to 5 days and can then be removed by saturating them with warm water, baby oil, or a small amount of liquid adhesive remover. Once the appliance is placed in the mouth, the retention tapes are connected to orthodontic elastics, which are then attached to the retention buttons on the base of the appliance and stretched over the base tape.

It is common for parents to feel anxious about the taping process. They need detailed instructions and ongoing support. Mastery of the process can take several weeks. Parents can call a member of the dental or orthodontic team at any time for advice. After the initial taping is completed, parents can take a photograph of their infant to use as a reference at home.

During the weekly or biweekly visits for assessment and appliance adjustment, the cleft team nurse will have many opportunities to monitor the baby's progress with feeding, weight gain, and overall growth and development. If the NAM therapy is being managed off-site (for example, in a dental or orthodontic office or clinic), the nurse specialist can call the parents periodically to offer advice and support. In some cases, a change of nipple or bottle will be indicated. Parents should encourage their child to use a pacifier during NAM therapy. The natural sucking motion will apply pressure on the gum ridges, which helps to mold them into the desired position. If a pacifier is used, it might need to be modified to better fit under the appliance. During these visits, the nurse can observe how the entire family is managing and can provide support as needed, especially as the date of the surgery approaches. A preoperative teaching session can be scheduled on the same day as one of the last appliance adjustments. Many parents need assurance that once the lip and alveolus are repaired, the baby will be able to adjust to feeding without the NAM appliance in place. The weekly or biweekly visits during NAM treatment provide parents with tremendous support and networking opportunities.

FEEDING A CLEFT-AFFECTED INFANT

Almost as soon as the cleft condition is diagnosed, parents have fears and concerns about feeding their infant. They may ask: "How will my baby eat?" "Won't food go into the nose and hurt him?" "Won't she choke when she eats?" "Will she be able to eat normal foods when she is older?" Emotions pertaining to their child's future can produce anxiety about feeding.

Feeding an infant with a cleft can be relatively straightforward with the proper feeding supplies and instructions. Some infants will have more complicated feeding problems and may need a feeding specialist. Different cleft teams may follow different feeding protocols, but their goal is similar: successful feeding.

Feeding Principles and Techniques

The normal feeding process involves coordinated sucking, swallowing, and breathing. Suction depends on the generation of negative pressure in a sealed oral cavity (the mouth) to draw the fluid from the nipple and into the mouth. A cleft makes it difficult for an infant to form the seals necessary to create these pressures. A cleft lip prevents a good seal around the nipple. A cleft palate prevents the child's ability to generate negative *intraoral* suction. Even small clefts of the soft palate and some submucosal clefts (which are often missed) can cause feeding problems.

Infants with clefts are at risk for a poor suck, air swallowing, milk entering the nose, long feeding times, and fatigue. These problems can cause poor weight gain.

Parents need a professional to provide early, consistent, and ongoing education and guidance to help them successfully feed their infant. This is often the role of the cleft team nurse specialist.

The following are important, common principles to refer to when feeding an infant with a cleft:
- Most infants with an isolated cleft lip or cleft lip and alveolus can generate appropriate suction and are able to breast-feed. Infants with a cleft palate will have an air leak through the cleft, which prevents effective suction on the breast or artificial nipple. Therefore most of these babies will not be able to obtain adequate nutrition through breast-feeding alone. (See Breast-Feeding for a more detailed discussion.)
- The bottle and feeding system chosen must allow the milk to flow easily. The flow should be adequate to keep the infant interested and awake, but slow enough to allow the infant to coordinate breathing between swallows.

- A free flow of milk allows less air to be swallowed. If a powdered formula is used, it should be stirred, not shaken.
- During feedings, babies may show signs of distress and discomfort. Parents need to recognize these signs, which include the following:
  - Pulling the head back and hyperextending the neck away from the bottle and nipple
  - A look of alarm, especially paired with a pause in the feeding rhythm or nasal escape of milk
  - Coughing or wet-sounding breathing
  - Waving, raising, or pushing the hands or arms on the bottle
  - Excessive blinking, eye widening, or frequent pauses in feeding
- The length of a feeding should be limited to 30 to 40 minutes. Longer feedings can cause exhaustion and require more energy, which prevents weight gain.
- The total volume of formula and/or breast milk intake should equal 5 to 7 ounces per kilogram of body weight per day (2.3 to 3.2 ounces per pound of body weight per day).
- The goal is to increase the baby's weight to the birth weight by approximately 2 weeks of age and to gain approximately 0.5 to 1 ounce per day.
- Parents should investigate their insurance coverage, because some will pay for specialty feeding bottles (under the category of medical supplies) and breast pumps. A written prescription or letter of medical necessity from the cleft team may improve the chances of successful insurance reimbursement.

In 2008 the Cleft Palate Foundation produced a comprehensive feeding video entitled *Feeding Your Baby,* written and produced by several professional team members of the American Cleft Palate-Craniofacial Association. It is available online *(www.cleftline.org)* in English, Spanish, and Chinese. The video is an excellent educational tool for parents and nurses who care for infants with a cleft lip and palate.

Step-by-Step Bottle-Feeding Instructions
The following list provides helpful instructions for feeding a cleft-affected baby:
1. Fill the bottle with more milk or formula than the infant can drink. This prevents the need to tip back the infant's head to swallow the last half ounce.
2. Place the infant in a semiupright position in good alignment and at 45 degrees or higher to decrease the milk coming through the nose (Fig. 7-2).
3. Tickle the corner of the mouth with the nipple or your finger, alerting the infant that the feeding will begin.
4. Wait for the infant's head to turn toward the nipple and the tongue to drop from the roof of the mouth.

5. Slip the nipple over the center of the tongue and wait for the infant to begin sucking. The baby's lips should begin to close around the nipple. Reposition the nipple so that the tip is in contact with an intact area of the palate. The bottle and nipple should be tipped downward, directing the milk away from the nose.

6. Observe the suck-swallow pattern. The infant should breathe every two to three swallows. Listen for an audible swallow, followed by a breath.

7. At first, some very young infants will suck and swallow many times and will not be able to stop to breathe. Remove the nipple until the infant catches his or her breath, and then reinsert it. Removing the nipple to decrease the flow is called *external pacing*. Most infants will develop better organization within a few days, often within a few feedings. Other ways to provide external pacing include tipping the bottle up so that the nipple does not fully fill; pulling the nipple to one side of the mouth to leave room at the edge for a breath; and, if using the SpecialNeeds Feeder (Haberman feeder), turning the nipple to the no-flow setting. The nipple should not be removed frequently unless the infant is not stopping to take a breath, because this will disrupt the infant's feeding rhythm.

8. Burp the infant after he or she has eaten approximately 1 ounce. Several methods can be used. The baby is seated and held upright on the parent's lap. The baby's chest and head are then tilted slightly forward. Alternatively, the infant can be positioned over the parent's shoulder. Often, all that is needed to elicit a burp is to straighten the infant's spine while lifting and supporting the chest and head.

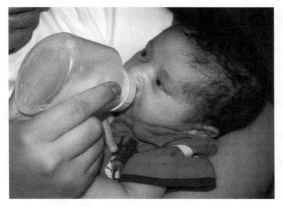

Fig. 7-2   This infant is held in a semiupright position for feeding.

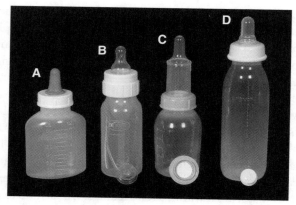

Fig. 7-3   **A,** Mead Johnson Cleft Lip/Palate Nurser. **B,** Dr. Brown's Specialty Feeding System. **C,** Medela SpecialNeeds Feeder (Haberman Feeder). **D,** Pigeon Specialty Feeding Cleft Palate Bottle.

Feeding Bottles and Nipples

Commonly used cleft feeding bottles and nipples are shown in Fig. 7-3.

Mead Johnson Cleft Lip/Palate Nurser

The Cleft Lip/Palate Nurser, commonly referred to as the Mead Johnson Bottle or the cleft squeeze bottle, is available in most newborn nurseries. The 6-ounce bottle has soft sides and can be easily squeezed (see Fig. 7-3, *A*). It comes packaged with a long, cross-cut nipple, although the nipple length and stiffness may be a problem for some infants. Many nurseries combine this bottle with a premature nipple or a standard single-hole nipple, depending on the needs of the infant.

When this bottle is used, squeezing should begin after the infant has begun sucking for a few seconds. The bottle is squeezed lightly initially, and then more heavily. Parents should watch the infant's face for distress signs. The testing process will reveal the rate of flow the infant can tolerate. The bottle is squeezed and released every two to three sucks. A stream of bubbles in the bottle after release indicates adequate compression.

The nipple should not be rubbed against the cleft, because this can cause irritation that progresses to a painful, reddened lesion.

Cleaning   The Mead Johnson Cleft Lip/Palate Nurser is marketed as a disposable bottle, which is how it is treated in the hospital. Once the baby is home, the bottle can be washed in hot, soapy water and is reusable for up to several weeks. It should not be sterilized, boiled, or placed in the dishwasher.

Dr. Brown's Specialty Feeding System

Dr. Brown's bottles are commercially available and frequently used for infants with gas or reflux (see Fig. 7-3, *B*). They have a patented, two-piece internal vent system. The company has developed a new bottle called the Dr. Brown's Specialty Feeding System. It consists of the Dr. Brown's Natural Flow bottle system with a one-way valve that fits into the nipple. The nipple is primed by squeezing it several times or by holding it at a 45-degree angle. Parents do not squeeze the bottle to feed the infant. Instead, the infant applies pressure to the nipple to make the milk flow. This bottle system can help to prevent gas issues common to infants with clefts.

The system is composed of either a 4-ounce or an 8-ounce bottle, a silicone nipple (with variable flow rates), and the Infant-Paced Feeding Valve. It is available for parents to purchase through major online retailers.

Dr. Brown's Specialty Feeding System is the newest of the specialty cleft bottles. It has received good reviews from specialists who have used it with cleft-affected babies.

Cleaning   Dr. Brown's bottle system is not disposable. The bottle, nipple, valve, and internal tube system can be boiled before the first use and regularly cleaned with hot, soapy water, in the top rack of the dishwasher, or with the microwave steam sterilizer bags.

SpecialNeeds Feeder (Haberman Feeder)

The SpecialNeeds Feeder (available for many years as the Haberman Feeder) was designed in the 1980s by Mandy Haberman, the mother of a child with Pierre Robin sequence. It is distributed by Medela, a company that manufactures breast pumps.

This feeder has four parts that can attach to most bottles (see Fig. 7-3, *C*). The soft silicone nipple has a slit-valve opening and a reservoir that holds approximately 27 milliliters of milk. Three line markings on the reservoir of the nipple indicate the position of the opening relative to the center of the baby's mouth. A white silicone valve is mounted to a polypropylene disc, and these are connected to a feeding bottle by a polypropylene collar. The feeding bottle is an 80- or 150-milliliter bottle that comes with the nipple.

This is a good feeder for an infant who requires a slower rate of flow or changes in the flow rate. To use this feeder, the bottle is filled with breast milk or formula. The assembled nipple-valve-disc-collar is attached to the bottle. To fill the nipple, the bottle is held upright and some air is squeezed out of the nipple. While the nipple is squeezed, the bottle is inverted and the nipple released. This is repeated until the nipple and reservoir are completely full.

Flow is controlled according to the direction of the slit in the nipple tip: no flow (smallest line), moderate flow (medium line) at 45 degrees, and high flow (long line) at 90 degrees. The nipple is inserted into the infant's mouth, with the smallest line on the nipple reservoir lined up with the center of the baby's nose; the nipple opening is at the horizontal, or zero flow, position. This gives the infant time to become adjusted to the nipple. Once sucking begins, the nipple can be rotated to increase the flow to a medium or high rate.

Many infants can activate and maintain an adequate flow rate on their own. However, the parent can squeeze the reservoir to assist the infant in increasing the flow of milk. Assistance with flow may require deep compression of the reservoir. Some parents prefer to compress the nipple with each jaw drop of the infant; others place pressure on the reservoir, releasing compression when the infant pauses.

Special considerations about the Medela SpecialNeeds Feeder include the following:
- A Mini SpecialNeeds Feeder is also available, providing a smaller-size nipple and reservoir for premature infants.
- This is the most expensive specialty feeder system. Parts of the bottle must be replaced on a regular basis. Because of the high cost, some parents will use another system.
- The multiple parts of the nipple can result in improper assembly and problems with successful use of the bottle.
- The bottle does not have a cover for the nipple and, because of its unusual appearance, often draws attention and questions from strangers.

Pigeon Specialty Feeding Cleft Palate Bottle

The Pigeon Feeder (see Fig. 7-3, *D*) is composed of an 8-ounce bottle; a wide, dual-thickness, vented, Y-cut nipple (in two sizes); and a one-way flow valve (placed in the base of the nipple). The nipple must be primed before it is placed in the infant's mouth. This is done by holding the filled bottle upright, squeezing the nipple, inverting the bottle, and releasing the nipple to allow it to fill with milk.

The thick side (the air valve side) of the nipple compresses against the hard palate. The soft, thin side of the nipple is placed above the tongue to promote optimal compression. When the thin side is compressed, milk is expressed into the infant's mouth. The air vent in the nipple base allows the nipple to refill with milk. The one-way valve prevents backflow of milk from the nipple into the bottle, thus helping to reduce the amount of air ingested during feeding.

This system allows the infant to control the flow of milk. Because the nipple is large, the parent should observe for signs of infant distress from too rapid a flow rate. If the infant swallows several times without taking a breath, rears the head back away from the nipple, or coughs, the flow may be too fast, and the nipple should be removed from the mouth (external pacing). Once the infant recovers, the nipple may be reinserted at a shallower angle to slow the flow of milk. The tightness of the collar also controls the milk flow. The tighter the collar, the slower the milk flow. Very young newborns will need some time to coordinate the rate of flow and should be watched closely for the first few feedings.

Special considerations about the Pigeon feeding system include the following:
- The Pigeon Bottle is sold with two nipples and valves, or a nipple and valve may be purchased separately. Nipples are available in two sizes: regular and small. The nipple and valve fit on most standard bottles. The valve can sometimes be used successfully in combination with other nipples, for example, fast-flow silicone nipples on vented bottles.
- Before a new nipple is used, it is necessary to roll the nipple tip between the fingers. The nipple has a tendency to collapse, slowing the flow of milk. This can be relieved by loosening the ring as it screws on the bottle. The triangular air vent needs to be dry, patent, and properly positioned under the infant's nose.

Cleaning   The nipple should be soaked and washed immediately after each feeding. The bottle can be washed with a bottle brush. The nipple, bottle, nipple ring, and flow valve should be boiled for 3 to 5 minutes after they are washed.

Breast-Feeding

The American Academy of Pediatrics and the U.S. Department of Health and Human Services recommend that infants from birth to 6 months of age be exclusively breast-fed. There are many reasons to choose human milk for an infant, particularly preterm infants, including the immunologic protection provided. Breast milk is well digested and less irritating to the palatal and nasal mucosa of an infant who may have frequent nasal regurgitation.

Babies with an isolated cleft of the lip should be able to adequately breast-feed. Some infants with a cleft lip and alveolus can lose partial suction through the cleft. In this case, the baby may need to be repositioned so that breast tissue fills the cleft. Alternatively, the cleft can be covered with a finger. The mother may need to hold

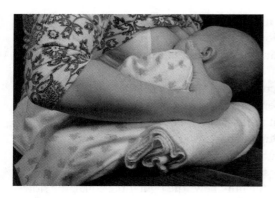

Fig. 7-4   This breast-feeding position is known as a modified football hold.

her breast in a position that pushes breast tissue into the gap. A feeding position with the infant facing the breast is sometimes needed in the first days of life to achieve a good seal (Fig. 7-4).

In rare cases, infants with a very small cleft of the soft palate or a bifid uvula can successfully breast-feed. However, most children with a cleft of the lip and palate and those with an isolated cleft of the hard and/or soft palate are not able to directly breast-feed exclusively. Most infants with a cleft palate are unable to create adequate intraoral suction and hold the nipple in place. Infants with a cleft palate who are beginning to breast-feed often require frequent feeding, supplemented with breast milk or formula. The mother must pump to maintain her milk supply. Newborn infants with a cleft who breast-feed need to be monitored closely for weight gain to prevent dehydration and weight loss. Parents should ask their care team for a list of signs of dehydration.

Tips for Breast-Feeding an Infant With a Cleft Palate

The following tips are for mothers who want to make a strong effort to directly and exclusively breast-feed their infant with a cleft palate:
- A lactation specialist should be sought for in-depth consultation and ongoing support.
- The mother must hold her breast in position throughout the feeding or the nipple will become dislodged. It is easier for a baby to latch on a nipple that is not flat.
- Some infants respond to a modified football hold or a straddle-hold position. The infant is sitting more upright, with the mouth facing the nipple. The

mother needs to support the baby on or against a pillow so that the mouth is even with the nipple.

- It may be helpful to stimulate letdown with manual expression or with the use of a breast pump before attempting to put the baby to the breast.
- The mother should pump after each feeding to maintain her milk supply. Ineffective nursing results in reduced stimulation to the breasts and decreased lactation.
- The inability to directly breast-feed may be very disappointing for a mother. But it is possible to put the baby to the breast after bottle-feeding to support bonding and to assist with letdown. A hospital or community lactation specialist can be very helpful in assisting with the purchase and use of a hospital-grade electric breast pump.

Tips for Expressing Breast Milk

- The use of a commercial electric pump is recommended. Hand pumping is not efficient enough for the volumes needed and the length of time required.
- Mothers should pump at least five to six times every day, saving the milk for a later feeding. Some mothers try to pump fresh milk but often feel too much stress when pumping while the baby is hungrily crying.
- To promote the most efficient milk production, the breasts should be massaged or warmed before pumping is started. Mothers can actively think about the baby while beginning to pump and try to relax.
- When the breast milk is inadequate for the whole feeding, all of the breast milk should be given before formula is added. This will prevent wasted breast milk should the infant not finish the bottle.
- If the breast milk supply seems inadequate, a consultation with a lactation consultant, obstetrician, or midwife may be helpful.
- Mothers should consult with the baby's pediatrician about the use of a human milk fortifier to help supplement the breast milk.
- If expressing milk becomes too stressful or if the supply is not adequate, it is perfectly acceptable and not harmful to the baby to supplement with or completely switch to formula.

Frequently Asked Questions About Feeding

How much should my baby eat?   A minimum intake of 2 ounces per pound of body weight in 24 hours is suggested. It can take up to a week to achieve this goal, depending on the condition of the child and the level of comfort of the parent.

How long should a feeding take?   Feedings should be limited to no more than 30 to 40 minutes. Feedings that last an hour or more usually indicate that an adjustment in the feeding method is needed. Premature infants are very difficult to keep awake and often require shorter, more frequent feedings.

How long can I let my baby sleep between feedings?   Infants in the first weeks of life should not sleep longer than 5 hours between feedings. If the baby is receiving breast milk, more frequent feedings may be needed, as often as every 2 to 3 hours. Once adequate fluid volumes and weight gain are achieved, the schedule can be relaxed to more of an on-demand feeding schedule.

Does my baby have acid reflux?   *Acid reflux,* also known as gastroesophageal reflux, is very common in all infants. It is particularly common in infants with a cleft palate, because they often swallow a large amount of air while eating. It may be helpful to elevate the head of the bed or to allow the infant to sit up for 30 minutes after eating. The primary care provider can be consulted about the baby's reflux symptoms, and if needed, a short course of acid-reducing medications may be given. If more severe symptoms occur, including pneumonia or poor weight gain, the mother and child can be referred to a gastroenterology specialist.

Will my baby choke when eating? What should I do if this happens?   It is important to differentiate choking from coughing that occurs after nasal regurgitation. It is common for babies with clefts of the palate to leak milk through the nose while being fed. If this happens, the feeding should be stopped and the baby positioned upward and forward. A nasal aspirator (bulb syringe), or preferably, a soft, damp cloth, can be used to gently clear the milk from the nose and mouth. After a short rest, the mother can resume feeding her baby. Choking or milk entering the lungs (aspiration) is extremely rare. If parents have any concerns about how the baby is managing feedings, they should consult with their pediatrician or cleft team nurse specialist.

When should my baby begin to eat solid foods?   The current recommendation of the American Academy of Pediatrics is to introduce solid foods when the child is 6 months of age. Parents can begin to spoon-feed thin solids with the baby in a slightly reclining position. They should begin with small amounts of rice cereal thinned with milk and should not become alarmed if some of the food comes out through the nose. They can begin with a teaspoon or two, morning and evening, and gradually increase the amount or the thickness of the food. When the consistency of the cereal is that of yogurt, parents can begin to add baby jar foods, one food group every 3 days, according to the preference of their pediatrician. A cup may be introduced when the baby is approximately 8 to 9 months of age to prepare for cup-feeding after the cleft palate repair. Parents can begin with thickened liquids from an open cup or a sippy cup with a recessed opening or a very short spout and the no-spill valve removed. Soft table foods may be introduced as recommended by the pediatrician. Parents need not be concerned about food entering the cleft areas. When fluids are given, food in the cleft will loosen and drain. In addition, the baby may automatically "sneeze out" any food stuck in the cleft. Parents can also use very gentle bulb syringe suctioning if needed, although this is rarely necessary.

CARING FOR A CHILD UNDERGOING CLEFT LIP REPAIR

The timing of cleft lip repair varies among teams, but usually occurs by 3 to 6 months of age (see Chapters 20 and 21). Parents should be familiar with the hospital's and the cleft team's postoperative routines. This information helps parents successfully care for their infant. Most hospitals offer programs providing general information and tours of the outpatient surgical suites and the inpatient pediatric units. The cleft team nurse can provide information about the postoperative period.

Parents' participation during their child's hospitalization is important. Parents should plan to be present as much as possible throughout the hospital stay, both in the postanesthesia care unit and in the hospital room if an overnight stay is needed. They may need to make arrangements for time off from work and, if necessary, changes to day care arrangements for the infant and siblings after surgery. Parents can look at photographs of other infants in the immediate postoperative period and talk with another family whose child has had the same surgery.

The goal of cleft lip surgery is to restore normal anatomy and function. Postoperative care routines are aimed at protecting the repair, minimizing pain, and maximizing the physical and psychological comfort of the infant.

Feeding

Depending on the cleft team surgeon, the infant may be allowed to breast-feed or to use the usual bottle immediately after surgery. If bottles are not allowed or the infant refuses the nipple, an alternative method may be required. A 30- to 60-milliliter syringe with a 1-inch rubber catheter tip or a manufactured soft squeeze bottle with thin tubing (for example, the TenderCare Feeder) can be used postoperatively. Parents can practice with the alternative method before surgery if they know that bottles will not be allowed after surgery. Pacifiers may not be allowed during this recovery period.

If the infant has been using a NAM appliance, the parents can practice feeding without the appliance in place before surgery. They can begin 1 to 2 weeks before the procedure, a few times a day. These infants are accustomed to having the appliance in place during feeding and may need time to readjust to feeding without it. The appliance is not needed for successful feeding.

Feedings are started once the baby is medically stable and is appropriately awake and alert. Clear fluids are offered first, and if the baby tolerates this, the feeding is progressed to full-strength breast milk or formula. Some teams allow a nursing infant to immediately return to the breast. Intravenous (IV) fluids are continued until the infant can tolerate adequate oral fluids. The IV rate can be decreased to increase the baby's thirst. Parents should ask their care team how much their infant will need to drink at home and monitor for signs of dehydration.

Elbow Splints

Removable splints may be required to keep the child's hands and other objects away from the repair site. This depends on the protocol of the cleft team. The splints can be removed for range of motion exercises and for skin inspection at regular intervals.

Incision Care

After surgery, the incision may need to be cleaned with saline solution on a cotton-tipped applicator or a small piece of gauze, and an antibiotic ointment may need to be applied. If the surgeon placed a *nasal stent,* the area around it will require gentle cleansing. When permanent (nonresorbable) sutures are used, they are removed 5 to 7 days postoperatively, either in the office or as a day surgery procedure. The child will be under anesthesia when the sutures are removed. Resorbable sutures and/or surgical glue may also be used. These do not need to be removed.

Pain Management

Postoperative pain is often difficult to assess in infants after cleft lip repair. The child may provide verbal and nonverbal cues, such as crying, restlessness, and body movements. Pain can be difficult to differentiate from irritability related to changes in the feeding method, the presence of restraints, nasal congestion, and the disruption of routines. To control pain, parents can hold and comfort their child, splints can be removed frequently, and nonnarcotic or narcotic pain medication can be given every 4 to 6 hours. Pain medication may be initially given through an IV line or rectally. As the infant begins to take fluids by mouth, oral medicine will be given (for example, acetaminophen, hydrocodone with acetaminophen, or oxycodone). Ibuprofen may not be recommended in the first few postoperative days because of the concern of possible increased bleeding.

Discharge From the Hospital

The hospitalization length may vary from that of an outpatient procedure to a 1-night inpatient stay. Discharge criteria usually include adequate fluid intake, observable pain control with oral medication, and the absence of a fever. Before discharge, parents need to understand and demonstrate the ability to care for the infant at home, including feeding, positioning, suture care, restraints, and giving medications. They may be instructed to continue to give pain medications every 4 to 6 hours for the first few postoperative days. After this time, most infants are comfortable without medication. Antibiotics are prescribed according to the team's protocol. Parents should be informed of the possible side effects (for example, rash, diarrhea, and oral thrush) and encouraged to contact the office if they observe these problems.

Parents are given contact telephone numbers of hospital personnel and team members to call any time of day or night with concerns or questions. They should report redness and drainage at the incision site, a temperature higher than 101° F (38.3° C), vomiting, diarrhea, decreased oral intake (or refusal to drink), and increasing or unrelieved pain. Follow-up appointments will be scheduled. Infants typically require 2 to 3 weeks to resume their preoperative routine, particularly if postoperative feeding restrictions and/or elbow restraints are needed.

Psychological and Emotional Issues

Parents who have anticipated surgery for many months often expect to be ecstatic when they see their baby after surgery. Many parents, however, have a difficult time adjusting to their infant's new appearance in the immediate postoperative period. They are not prepared for such conflicting feelings. Some are distressed at the first glance of their child in the postanesthesia care unit, stating that the child does not look like their baby. These feelings usually pass quickly as parents get used to the new lip repair. Some parents are also very anxious about assuming immediate responsibility for the baby's postoperative care, especially if the surgery is performed on an outpatient basis.

CARING FOR A CHILD UNDERGOING CLEFT PALATE REPAIR

Palate repair (palatoplasty) is usually performed when the child is 9 to 12 months of age, depending on factors such as the type of cleft, the surgeon's preference, and the child's weight and overall health. The goal of surgery is to establish normal palatal function before the onset of speech development (see Chapter 23).

Feeding

Swelling and discomfort during swallowing may delay the start of oral feeds. Pain medication is given promptly so that the infant does not associate pain with drinking. Oral feeds may begin when the child is fully awake and is medically stable. Offering small amounts of liquids at frequent intervals is helpful. Dietary restrictions are usually in place for 1 to 3 weeks; good hydration is emphasized during this time. As with the cleft lip repair, postoperative feeding restrictions are based on the cleft team's preferences.

Depending on the age of the child, transitioning to cup-feeding before surgery is helpful. Although some surgeons allow the use of a bottle postoperatively, most children undergoing palate repair are old enough to begin the weaning process. The use of cups with spouts may or may not be allowed postoperatively. Straws and utensils should not be used. Parents should ask their team to explain their specific requirements. Some centers prescribe a progressive diet, starting with clear liquids and progressing to liquefied foods (for example, stage 1 or 2 jar foods with added water or blenderized table foods) that can be fed with a spoon held parallel to the lips. Water should be offered after feedings, because it can help to cleanse the mouth and will minimize the child's tendency to attempt to clear the palate with the tongue. It is helpful for parents to have a specific, written feeding protocol so that they can plan accordingly.

Airway Management

After the palate is repaired, care involves protecting the repair, monitoring the infant for excessive bleeding, and monitoring the airway. Postoperative swelling of the palate and/or tongue and thick secretions and drainage can occur. Infants are usually monitored overnight with a pulse oximeter. A nasopharyngeal airway may be left in place, particularly in children with Pierre Robin sequence. A tongue suture can be inserted in the operating room before the child is awake; it is taped to the cheek for use if the child has airway problems. Pulling downward on the tongue stitch to reposition the tongue can relieve obstruction. The appearance of this suture can be frightening to parents; it is helpful for them to view a picture of it preoperatively. The infant can be placed on the stomach to promote drainage of secretions.

Splints and Behavioral Issues

Elbow splints may be required to keep the infant's hands, toys, and other objects out of the mouth. Older infants may be more adept at removing these restraints. The child can wear a long-sleeve shirt with the cuffs pulled over the splints to prevent removal. Alternatively, the splints can be pinned to the child's clothes.

Because of their developmental stage, children having palate repair may have more difficulty adapting to limitations on diet and activity. They can be irritable and difficult to console. Parents should be aware of this so that they can anticipate the behavioral changes and manage with less anxiety.

Discharge From the Hospital

The hospital stay after palate repair is usually 1 to 2 days, typically a little longer than that required for lip repair, because children at this stage can be willful and refuse to take anything by mouth. Discharge criteria include comfortable breathing, adequate fluid intake, and effective pain control with oral medication. Discharge instructions include diet and feeding instructions, the use of restraints, and instructions for giving pain medication. Parents are usually instructed to report a fever higher than 101° F (38.3° C), bleeding and drainage from the palate, inadequate fluid intake, refusal to drink, vomiting, diarrhea, and excessive crying or pain unrelieved by medication.

CARING FOR A CHILD UNDERGOING ALVEOLAR BONE GRAFTING

The timing of alveolar bone grafting to repair the alveolar cleft is based on the child's dental development and the recommendation of the orthodontist. This surgery is typically performed when the child is 6 to 12 years of age to support the healthy eruption of the permanent teeth into the cleft site. Although bone can be taken from several donor sites, it is usually taken from the iliac crest (hip) (see Chapter 29).

Preoperative preparation is needed for the school-age child and the parents. At this age, children are able to understand information about surgery, the preoperative evaluation, and postoperative changes in their routine. They should be encouraged to ask questions about all aspects of the surgery, hospital stay, and the postoperative activity restrictions. This is especially important for children who participate in sports. Networking with another child of the same age who has completed this surgery can be very helpful. Medical play with a child life specialist may allow children to work through fears about surgery and separation. Rarely, a child will develop extreme anxiety about medical treatment, and referral to a therapist is indicated. A nutrition consultation can be helpful for planning the postoperative diet.

Postoperative care is aimed at protecting both the graft (bone that is transferred to the gum) and the donor site (usually the hip). Both areas need to be observed for bleeding and signs of infection. IV fluids are continued until oral fluids are tolerated.

Feeding

Clear liquids are offered as soon as the child is alert and able to swallow; the diet is progressed to blenderized or soft foods, according to the protocol of the child's cleft team. The child can be given oral liquid supplements to help maximize caloric intake. Utensils and straws should be placed inside the mouth carefully to prevent injury to the graft site. A nutrition consultation (either preoperatively or before the child is discharged from the hospital) can be very helpful to the family. A written explanation of the diet restrictions, with examples of allowable foods, should be reviewed with the child and parents. These restrictions may need to be followed for up to 8 weeks. Oral hygiene includes mouth rinses with water or a prescription mouthwash. Careful brushing of the upper teeth can begin once the graft site is healed, but the lower teeth and tongue can be brushed immediately after surgery. Depending on the center, a dental splint may be inserted for up to 8 to 12 weeks.

Pain Management

Pain is initially managed with IV narcotics in the immediate postoperative period. This very effectively manages pain in these children and can be used until they tolerate oral fluids. Oral pain medication can then be given, either a liquid preparation or a crushed tablet.

The iliac bone graft site is generally closed with absorbable sutures and covered with a waterproof dressing. Discomfort is often greater at the iliac crest harvest site than in the mouth. Pain medication given 20 to 30 minutes before ambulation may be helpful. Elevation of the head and/or the application of ice packs can improve facial swelling, which can be significant, especially in a child who requires bilateral alveolar grafts.

Discharge From the Hospital

Alveolar bone grafting may be performed as an outpatient procedure or may require an overnight stay, depending on the protocol of the cleft team and the patient's postoperative progress. Discharge instructions should include information on diet, medication administration, bathing, oral hygiene, care of the bone graft site, return to school, and activity restrictions. Tub bathing can resume once the incision at the donor site is completely healed. The child may be slow to ambulate, and climbing stairs can be difficult for a few days. Cleft team–specific restrictions for activities such as contact sports, bike-riding, and skateboarding are reviewed with the child and family. The school should be informed of diet and activity restrictions, including nonparticipation in gym class and recess.

CARING FOR A CHILD UNDERGOING SECONDARY PALATAL SURGERY

School-age children with velopharyngeal dysfunction (see Chapter 12) may require additional surgical management. Preoperative evaluation can include a complete speech evaluation, a sleep study (see Chapter 17), and *videofluoroscopy* or *nasoendoscopy*. A tonsillectomy may be indicated and is usually performed at least 6 weeks before secondary palatal surgery. Nurses will help to inform and prepare the child and family for the evaluation procedures.

Postoperative management for surgical procedures to treat velopharyngeal dysfunction is similar to that after a palatoplasty. Potential complications after surgery are bleeding and/or airway obstruction. The nasal airway may be reduced in size and compromised by postoperative swelling. Close monitoring for signs of airway obstruction is necessary.

Feeding

The use of straws and utensils may be restricted after surgery. A blenderized or soft food diet is usually necessary for 2 to 3 weeks, along with careful oral hygiene practices. A nutrition consultation can provide creative solutions for the school-age child's diet preferences.

Pain Management

Oropharyngeal (mouth and throat) pain and neck pain are common; some children are reluctant to even swallow their saliva. Children may also be irritable and may be hesitant to speak immediately after surgery because of discomfort or fear. Adequate pain management is critical in encouraging the school-age child to drink. Before the child is discharged, IV narcotics are discontinued. Parents can give oral medications at home.

Discharge From the Hospital

Discharge instructions are similar to those given after the initial palate repair. In addition, information about observation for obstructive sleep apnea should be given to the parents (see Chapter 17).

CONCLUSION

The nurse on the cleft team plays an integral role in educating and supporting the family and the patient from birth to maturity and serves as the patient's and family's liaison to the rest of the cleft team. Feeding the infant with a cleft is often one of the most difficult parts of a parent's experience, and this is one of the areas in which the team nurse's expertise is particularly valuable. For parents of a child with Pierre Robin sequence, the team nurse is an essential resource for learning about healthy breathing patterns and safe feeding techniques. The team nurse also helps to optimize surgical outcomes and makes surgery easier for the patient and the family, guiding them through perioperative care.

8

The Role of the Pediatrician in Cleft Care

Rachel Harmon, Dawn Leavitt, Michael L. Cunningham

KEY POINTS

- The pediatrician is at the center of the cleft-affected child's care, beginning with prenatal involvement through adolescence.

- Soon after the child's birth, ideally the team pediatrician will conduct a thorough physical examination and a complete assessment of the cleft. Babies with a cleft palate are often unable to breast-feed; therefore feeding may need to be adjusted for optimal growth.

- The lip is typically repaired when the child is 3 to 6 months of age. The pediatrician will have regular contact with the infant and family to answer the parents' questions and to ensure that the infant is ready for the surgery.

- The cleft palate is usually repaired when the child is 9 to 15 months of age. The pediatrician will continue to focus on preparing the child for palate surgery and assessing the infant's growth and development.

- After the palate repair, as the infant enters toddlerhood, the preschool years, and the transition to adulthood, the pediatrician monitors other areas, including speech and hearing and dental, social, and psychological factors.

Some cleft centers do not have a pediatrician on their team and rely on the community primary care provider to ensure the general well-being of cleft-affected children. Specialized pediatricians who are members of cleft center teams play an important role in the long-term care of these patients. The pediatrician is at the center of the child's care, working as a liaison between the child and family and the other interdisciplinary care providers. The pediatrician informs the other care providers about the patient's unique needs and facilitates their involvement in the treatment, while helping the patient and parents understand the various providers' recommendations. During each visit, the pediatrician medically evaluates the patient and gathers information about the family's values, beliefs, and preferences. Through ongoing collaboration with the cleft or craniofacial team and the family, the pediatrician can provide the best care for the patient. Throughout the patient's childhood and adolescence, the pediatrician has the following responsibilities:

- Coordination of the patient's lip, palate, and nose surgeries
- Management of issues related to growth and development (including speech and hearing)
- Promotion of the patient's dental care and health
- Assessment of the patient's psychosocial adjustment

This chapter will discuss the specific duties of the pediatrician during the various stages of childhood and adolescence.

PRENATAL INVOLVEMENT

With today's advanced technology, clefts are commonly diagnosed in an ultrasound evaluation between 18 and 40 weeks of pregnancy (see Chapter 6). When a prenatal diagnosis of a cleft is made, the parents usually receive a referral to a cleft and craniofacial center for additional information. The first meeting with the team will help the parents understand the diagnosis and begin to prepare for their child's care. Parents will learn specific information about their child, based on the information provided in the ultrasound evaluation. For instance, the parents may learn about differences between a *unilateral cleft* and a *bilateral cleft* and the differences between a cleft lip and a cleft palate. Additional evaluations might be recommended to gather more diagnostic information. Examples of other evaluations include a fetal echocardiogram (heart ultrasound examination to determine whether heart problems are present) and genetic counseling to better understand the likelihood of a genetic syndrome (see Chapter 5).

Parents often have a range of emotions, including shock, grief, loss, guilt, anger, and fear. During the initial meeting, the pediatrician works to build a rapport with the parents by validating their feelings, listening to their concerns and questions, and asking about their beliefs and support systems. Additional supportive services may be recommended. For families with a limited support system, the pediatrician will want to know of possible difficulties seeking care after the child is born; the team can help to minimize or eliminate some of these barriers.

In addition, parents will learn what to expect when the child is born and may meet other members of the interdisciplinary team. For example, a child with a cleft palate will likely not be able to breast-feed. The pediatrician or the team feeding expert will discuss feeding options and additional information about specialized bottles and pumping milk. At these visits, a social worker may be present to provide emotional support and links to additional resources. (See Chapters 7 and 11 for more details about the role of these professionals on the cleft or craniofacial team.)

The prenatal visits should help families feel more prepared to care for their baby. They will receive information about what happens at birth and possible postnatal complications that are not identified on ultrasound evaluations. These include respiratory (breathing) problems, hearing issues, and learning disabilities. At the end of these visits, families will be told when to return for their first visit with their new baby.

BIRTH

Physical Examination

When a child with a cleft is born, ideally the team pediatrician will meet the infant within the first week. At the first visit, the pediatrician will thoroughly examine the baby to assess the cleft. Parents will find out whether the cleft involves the lip, the palate, or both; whether the cleft is unilateral or bilateral; and whether it is *complete* or *incomplete*. Additional tests will be performed if other health concerns are possible, such as heart issues or genetic conditions. Hearing is assessed at birth, because children with clefts can have hearing loss (see Chapters 14 and 15). The pediatrician also assesses the infant's ability to breathe adequately.

Growth

Adequate growth is essential during the first weeks of life. The team will focus on growth to ensure that the infant is thriving in preparation for surgery. Because babies with a cleft palate are likely not able to breast-feed, their feeding schedule is adjusted. At the first visit, the baby will be weighed to establish a baseline weight, assess how the baby is feeding, and inform the feeding specialist about any difficulties. Care providers will help parents find an appropriate bottle. If the mother wants to feed her child breast milk, she will learn how to use a breast pump. The pediatrician will gather information about the family's preferences and concerns and share it with other team members to help them better prepare for working with the family.

Preparation for Surgery

The pediatrician will begin to prepare the parents for the infant's lip repair surgery. Some infants need presurgical treatments such as nasoalveolar molding, lip adhesion, or taping techniques (see Chapters 27 and 28). The pediatrician will introduce the parents to the orthodontist and surgeon. The goal of these treatments is to decrease the size of the cleft and optimize the surgical outcome. The use of orthodontic devices requires a large commitment from the family, including frequent visits and daily care for the device; therefore the team assesses the family's ability and desire to take part in this process.

FIRST FIVE MONTHS

Preparation for Lip Repair

After the first visit, the team will recommend when to return. This depends on the complexity of the cleft and the health of the patient. Throughout the first few months, the pediatrician will have regular contact with the patient and family to ensure that the patient is ready for the first lip repair. This surgery usually is performed when the child is 3 to 6 months of age. Areas of focus include growth and feeding, other health difficulties, and the patient's and family's coping with and adjustment to orthodontic devices. The patient's heart and lungs will be examined thoroughly, because anesthesia will be given during the lip repair surgery. The team members will talk with the family about what to expect after the lip repair. Some parents are surprised that it takes time to adjust to the appearance of their child's repaired cleft.

The patient and family will meet various medical providers during these early weeks. The parents will benefit from understanding the roles of each one. The pediatrician communicates with the surgeon, orthodontist, social worker, nurses, and community providers about the family's and patient's challenges and continues to provide emotional support for the parents, who are adapting to caring for their child.

TRANSITION TO TODDLERHOOD: FIVE TO FIFTEEN MONTHS OF AGE

During the baby's first 5 to 15 months of age, the family will continue to see the pediatrician. The focus during this period is preparation for palate surgery (if needed) and the infant's growth and development. The cleft palate is typically repaired when the child is 9 to 15 months of age.

Developmental Milestones

The pediatrician tracks the child's progress in meeting developmental milestones and determines whether additional services or evaluations can be beneficial. These include early intervention services for physical, feeding, and occupational therapy. Children with clefts can be at risk for developmental delay because of poor growth from feeding difficulties, hearing loss, speech problems, and associated syndromes.

Nutrition

The care provider will continue to track feeding habits and ensure that the infant is growing well. Many infants begin to eat solid foods during this time. In infants with a cleft palate, food can pass through the palate and exit through the nose. The pediatrician will prepare caregivers for this possibility. Infants having continued difficulty gaining or maintaining weight may need help from a nutritionist and/or feeding specialist before the palate is repaired.

Ears

Infants with a cleft palate often have ear-related problems such as fluid in the ears, recurrent ear infections, and hearing difficulties (see Chapters 14 and 15). Parents will share information about their child's ear infections and discuss their concerns about the child's hearing. Most children can participate in a behavioral hearing screen after they are 7 months of age. For children with recurrent ear infections, middle-ear fluid, and/or decreased hearing, the otolaryngologist may recommend ear tubes. These are often placed during the palate surgery.

Respiratory Health

Some cleft-affected infants have breathing difficulties. The pediatrician will ask the parents about the child's history of cough, wheezing, and respiratory distress and assess for any signs of respiratory distress. This information is needed to prepare for the cleft palate repair.

Dental Health

An infant's teeth will start to come in during this time. Children with clefts may be missing teeth or have teeth that are not properly aligned. They have a higher risk of poor dental health, in part because of the placement of the teeth and difficulty brushing them. The care provider will begin to educate the family about the importance of good oral hygiene. The child may be referred to a dentist. Good oral health will help to increase the success of future orthodontic treatments and surgeries.

Preparation for Surgery

The surgeon will answer parents' questions about the upcoming palate repair and provide guidance about what to expect after the surgery. The family can share experiences regarding the lip repair and how these may be influencing their thoughts and feelings about the next surgery.

LATE TODDLERHOOD AND PRESCHOOL YEARS

After the palate repair is completed, the focus of care includes speech and language development. The pediatrician continues to monitor the child's cognitive development and physical development and all other health issues. During this period, the child will prepare for starting kindergarten. Some children require additional surgeries during this stage, such as a surgery involving a lip or a nose revision.

Speech and Hearing

Many cleft-affected children need speech and language therapy because of the anatomy of their palate. The speech and language are evaluated, and a referral for ongoing speech therapy is provided as needed. The goal is to ensure that the child's speech is understandable when he or she starts elementary school.

Toddlers and preschoolers will continue to undergo hearing tests regularly. Providers will continue to monitor for ear infections and the need for ear tubes.

Dental Health

The pediatrician will emphasize the importance of maintaining good oral hygiene and look for any signs of cavities or poor gum health. If the parents need additional instructions, the team will provide them or refer the family to a dentist.

Social and Psychological Issues

Parents should share their concerns about their child's behaviors at home or preschool. The pediatrician will ask about stressors that might be affecting the family and issues regarding the cleft that have occurred in social settings. Parents considering having another child may want to discuss the risks for the recurrence of clefts.

SCHOOL AGE

After the child enters school, the pediatrician will evaluate social and emotional adjustments and any concerns that arise as a result of having a cleft. Medically, the focus is on oral health and preparation for alveolar bone grafting. The care provider begins to encourage the child to participate during visits and to ask questions about the cleft and overall health.

School Readiness

The pediatrician will determine whether the child has developmental delays that can affect school readiness and refer for additional services as needed.

Social and Psychological Issues

As children progress through elementary school, they usually become more aware of their facial difference. Peers begin to notice and may comment and ask questions. The pediatrician and team social worker or psychologist can support the child and parents by assisting them in formulating answers and by addressing the child's concerns. Additional psychosocial support might be helpful for children and families having many difficulties. For children with possible learning challenges, providers will ask about any academic problems that occur at school.

Dental Health

Good oral health continues to be critical to the school-age child's well-being. During this developmental stage, cleft-affected children will have ongoing orthodontist visits as their mouth and jaw develop and adult teeth begin to come in. The orthodontic team, dentist, and surgeon discuss the child's oral health and the timing of the alveolar bone graft. The medical specialists will pay particular attention to the child's dental *occlusion*.

Speech and Hearing

Many children with a cleft palate will continue to have ear infections and require ear tubes. They should continue to have regular hearing tests. Velopharyngeal insufficiency or dysfunction can be identified at this time. The pediatrician will work with the speech-language therapist, surgeon, and otolaryngologist to determine whether a speech device or surgery would help to resolve this issue (see Chapter 12).

Sleep Apnea

Sleep apnea can be associated with a cleft in the lip, nose, and/or palate (orofacial cleft). The pediatrician, otolaryngologist, and other team members will screen for symptoms of *obstructive sleep apnea* by asking parents questions about their child's snoring, decreased school performance, or daytime fatigue.

ADOLESCENCE

Adolescence is an important time, when teenagers work to become more independent from the adults in their lives. For a child with a cleft, adolescence is an opportunity to increase autonomy in medical decision-making. Adolescents tend to focus more on appearance; the presence of a facial difference can present unique challenges for a young person's self-image.

School and Psychosocial Adjustment

The team providers focus on the teenager's questions and specific concerns about his or her facial difference. Some adolescents may worry about their appearance and desire additional lip and nose reconstruction or repair of their *midface hypoplasia*. Others may worry about speech or orthodontic issues. Providers should talk openly with teenage patients, empowering them to make their own decisions.

Often, teenagers and their parents disagree over the next steps in medical care. The parents may want their child to have additional surgery on the lip or nose, whereas the child may be comfortable with his or her facial appearance. The pediatrician provides the teenager with all of the information needed to make educated decisions and informs other team members about the patient's social situation and goals.

Adolescents will be screened for risky behaviors (for example, drug use) and mental health status during visits to care providers and will receive referrals to psychosocial professionals as needed for extra support.

Surgery

During the adolescent years, some patients are interested in additional lip or nose revisions. *Orthognathic surgery* is often recommended for adolescents with midface hypoplasia.

Dental

The care provider will assess the patient's dental health and hygiene and consult with the orthodontist and dentist as needed. Some teenagers benefit from braces.

Genetics

Adolescence is an important time to begin to discuss genetics and the risk of cleft recurrence. Many teenagers start to wonder if their children will have clefts and may be referred to the team's geneticist or genetic counselor.

TRANSITION TO ADULT CARE: EIGHTEEN TO TWENTY-ONE YEARS OF AGE

As adolescents approach adulthood, the pediatrician will provide them with referrals to medical professionals who work specifically with adults and provide the information they need to make this transition. Teenagers typically have a variety of feelings about transitioning from the pediatrician who has, in many cases, known and helped them their whole life.

CONCLUSION

A child with a cleft has unique medical needs that require careful collaboration among the patient, parents, and a variety of medical providers. The pediatrician, whether primary care or part of a cleft team, is instrumental in this process. This provider plays a central role in educating the patient and family throughout their journey and in facilitating an individualized and comprehensive care approach from the interdisciplinary team.

Part II

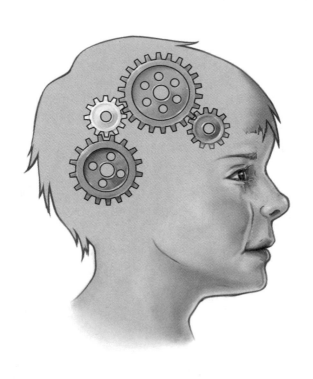

Psychosocial and Educational Aspects of Cleft Care

Psychological and Behavioral Considerations

Canice E. Crerand, Celia E. Heppner

KEY POINTS

○ Parents can help their preschool-age child cope effectively and develop resilience by forming bonds with their child through nondirected play time, by monitoring their own stress about their child's difference, through early education about cleft lip or palate (CLP), and by rehearsing appropriate responses to questions from peers.

○ Parents can help their school-age child cope effectively and develop resilience by providing opportunities for socialization and development of peer relationships, by staying in touch with the craniofacial team as their child grows and is able to better communicate needs and desires, and by helping to develop a positive body image.

○ Parents can help their child during adolescence and teenage years to cope effectively and develop resilience by encouraging an active role in health care, by teaching critical thinking about media images of appearance ideals, and by engaging a mental health professional if their child shows signs of depression related to his or her appearance.

○ Many support systems are available for families through craniofacial teams and support organizations.

The American Cleft Palate-Craniofacial Association's *Parameters of Care for the Evaluation and Treatment of Patients With Cleft Lip/Palate* specifies that craniofacial teams should have a specialist who can assist families with *psychosocial* needs. These services may look quite different from clinic to clinic, with some teams offering psychosocial evaluation and services as part of children's regular team visits, and others offering referrals to providers outside of the clinic. Mental health providers within clinics include psychologists, social workers, clinical therapists, and psychiatrists. These professionals can monitor the patients' psychological functioning throughout their treatment. They can also provide support and guidance to parents to help them cope with the child's condition. Finally, they can help to ensure that the cleft-affected child gains access to resources such as early intervention services for speech therapy and learning support services at school.

The goals of this chapter are to help parents learn about some of the potential challenges associated with raising a child with CLP and to highlight ways that they can help their child meet these challenges. Several points are important to emphasize. First, every child, with or without a cleft, faces challenges, and not every child with a cleft will have psychosocial problems related to their difference. Second, a relatively large amount of research is available about the psychological effects of CLP; this work shows that most cleft-affected children are remarkably resilient and do not have significant emotional or behavioral problems. Research has also found that most young adults who were treated for CLP as children are able to acknowledge that their experience shaped their lives and personalities in positive ways. However, each case is unique. Whereas some children have few problems, others may have more difficulties. Challenges are highlighted here because these are the concerns that tend to be most worrisome for parents, and being aware of these risks can help parents take an active role in intervening early should problems occur. Recommendations for at-risk children aim to promote resilience and positive coping throughout childhood and adolescence.

In this chapter, we describe the types of challenges that families may encounter, from common reactions to learning about a child's diagnosis through concerns that can arise during early adulthood. Each section offers suggestions for how parents

Box 9-1   Helpful Organizations

Name	Website
Ameriface	*http://www.ameriface.org/*
Changing Faces	*https://www.changingfaces.org.uk/*
Children's Craniofacial Association (CCA Kids)	*http://www.ccakids.org/*
Cleft Palate Foundation	*http://www.cleftline.org/*
Wide Smiles	*http://www.widesmiles.org/*
Zero-to-Three	*http://www.zerotothree.org/*

can support their child and effectively address common problems. Box 9-1 lists organizations that provide support and information for families of children with CLP. Parents are encouraged to talk with their craniofacial team coordinator, team psychologist, and social worker about local and hospital-based support programs for children and families (see Chapter 1).

COPING WITH A CHILD'S CLEFT CONDITION: CHALLENGES AND OPPORTUNITIES

Learning About the Child's Diagnosis

Because prenatal ultrasound examinations are routinely performed throughout pregnancy for most mothers, families usually learn of their child's cleft before the child is born. However, some children are diagnosed with a cleft at birth. Whether the diagnosis is made prenatally or at birth, learning that their infant has a cleft is usually a surprise to families. Feelings of worry, sadness, and guilt are common responses. Many parents wonder if they did something to cause their child's cleft. CLP is caused by a variety of factors; genetics play a large role, and in most cases, the cleft is not caused by something a parent did or did not do. An important first step for parents after finding out that their infant has a cleft is to seek education about CLP and its treatment. This information often helps parents cope with worries and uncertainty related to their child's treatment. After a diagnosis is made, families can (and should) seek out and meet with their craniofacial team members to ask questions and develop a treatment plan. Face-to-face and online support groups are also available in many communities (see Box 9-1).

Parents may find it difficult to tell friends and family about their child's diagnosis. Sharing this news and providing them with basic information about the condition and treatment can help others to understand what parents and infants with CLP are experiencing. Support from friends, extended family, and people in the community (for example, neighbors and members of the parents' place of worship) also helps parents cope with the normal stressors of having a new baby with a facial difference. For families with other children, talking to the cleft-affected child's siblings about the new baby's diagnosis of CLP can be challenging. For younger children, simple, straightforward explanations tend to be best (for example, "Your little sister has a cleft lip, which means she will be born with a split in her lip. She'll have surgery to close the split when she's a few months old."). Siblings can also benefit from looking at photos of infants with unrepaired clefts in preparation for seeing their sibling for the first time.

Infancy and Preschool Years

Attachment is a critical part of early development for all infants. During the first year of life for an infant with CLP, developing a healthy, secure bond is the most important thing a parent can do to promote healthy psychological functioning throughout childhood. A common concern for parents of children with CLP is whether being unable to breast-feed will affect attachment. It is definitely possible to develop a healthy attachment when breast-feeding is not an option. Maintaining skin-to-skin and eye contact during feeds, being responsive to the baby's needs, and maintaining a consistent, predictable schedule are all important activities that promote secure attachment.

Given the feeding difficulties, frequent medical appointments, and multiple surgical procedures, the first year of life can be stressful for parents of a child with CLP. Research suggests that a cleft-affected child will have fewer behavioral and social problems later in childhood if the parents (especially the mother) manage stress well during the child's infancy. Stress can affect parents' functioning and cause them to feel more anxious, easily frustrated, and sadder than normal, in addition to causing changes in their appetite and energy level. Parents may better manage these stressors by relying on social support and coping strategies that worked well in the past (for example, taking time to do a fun activity, exercising, and using relaxation strategies such as deep breathing or meditation).

During the child's early childhood and preschool years, psychological providers on craniofacial teams typically focus on evaluating developmental milestones. They provide recommendations when the child is not meeting milestones as expected. Delays in speech development are common for young children with CLP, but other developmental delays can also be seen. If parents are concerned about their child's development, it is important for them to talk with their team psychologist so that early intervention services can be initiated. Parents of young children with CLP often become very focused on ensuring that their child is gaining developmental skills. Although it is important for parents to be proactive about intervention for developmental skills, nondirected play time is also critical for social and emotional development in young children and preschoolers. Parents who have a young child involved in many directive, structured activities (for example, speech and other developmental therapies) can help their child develop important social and emotional skills by dedicating as little as 10 to 15 minutes of time each day to free play, in which the child chooses how he or she plays.

Many parents of children with facial differences have concerns about sending their child to preschool. Preschool is an important social experience for young children and can help to prepare them to be successful in kindergarten. A common worry for parents is that their child will be teased by peers because of his or her appearance. At this age, bullying is less common; however, many preschool children with CLP report that peers ask them questions about their appearance. Although these questions tend to be more curiosity based than intentionally unkind, preschoolers can sometimes be distressed or uncomfortable when asked why they look different. Preparing and rehearsing an age-appropriate response to appearance-related questions can help children with CLP feel more comfortable responding and increases their self-confidence and understanding of their facial difference.

What Parents Can Do to Promote Resilience

Parents can help their infant or preschool-age child develop resilience in many ways, including:
- Helping to develop a secure, healthy attachment with their baby by being affectionate, nurturing, and responsive to his or her needs.
- Paying attention to their own stress and seek help if it seems to be affecting them negatively. Their primary care doctor or the craniofacial team's psychologist can provide more recommendations for help with managing stress.
- Monitoring their child's development. Information about promoting healthy development in young children is available through the Zero to Three Center.
- Enjoy playtime with their infant or young child. Play is a critical part of early development.
- Beginning to educate their child about the cleft when he or she is young. They should be open about discussing the diagnosis. Children look to their parents for cues about how to think and feel about their cleft; therefore it should not be discussed as a negative or shameful difference. Taking pho-

tos of the infant before and after surgery is encouraged. The child can look at these pictures to better understand the cleft on entering early childhood and school age.

- Helping their preschooler rehearse an age-appropriate response to questions about his or her appearance. A brief, clear explanation ("I was born with a split in my lip, and my doctor fixed it.") tends to work best for children in this age group, followed by steering the conversation in a different direction ("Want to play with this toy?").

School-Age Children

Entering school can be both an exciting and an anxious time for children and their parents. School offers children opportunities to learn, develop new skills, become more independent, and establish friendships and interests. On the other hand, parents may worry about how others will view and treat their child, particularly if the child has a facial difference or speech difficulties. Parents may also wonder if their child's cleft will affect his or her ability to learn and succeed at school. Another stressor families might face during this stage is preparing the child for additional cleft-related surgeries to improve speech and/or appearance.

Siblings of children with CLP can also have worries and concerns. Some fear being teased because of their sibling's differences. They can be jealous of the attention that their cleft-affected sibling receives from their parents. In some instances, these worries can affect family dynamics. For example, parents who are anxious sometimes try to protect children from situations in which their differences may be noticed. However, overprotection can result in children missing opportunities to develop confidence in social situations and can make children more self-conscious and anxious in the long term.

Research on school-age children with CLP suggests that they generally have normal intelligence and do not develop emotional, behavioral, or social difficulties. However, they have a slightly elevated risk of intellectual disabilities, approximately 4% to 6% of children with CLP have intellectual disabilities, compared with just 2% of children from the general population. They also have an increased risk of learning disabilities related to language, reading, and memory; approximately 30% to 40% of children with CLP have a learning disability. A learning disability can affect a child's behavior, emotional functioning, and relationships with peers. For example, children who have difficulty with learning can have more problems paying attention or following directions in the classroom. They might think about themselves negatively, having thoughts such as "I'm not smart." This can in turn affect self-esteem and mood.

Studies suggest that children with CLP are at risk for social problems such as shyness, withdrawing from peer interaction, and teasing. Some can develop a low *self-concept,* meaning that they are more likely to negatively evaluate aspects of themselves such as their intelligence, self-worth, and appearance. Children with a low self-concept can be more vulnerable to bullying. Some children with CLP feel self-conscious about their appearance and/or speech, although studies suggest that there are few differences in how children with and without the condition rate their appearance. Given society's emphasis on appearance, a degree of dissatisfaction with appearance is common among all children.

What Parents Can Do to Promote Resilience

Parents can help their school-age child develop resilience in many ways, including:

- Talking with their child's craniofacial team members about speech, appearance, learning, and behavior concerns. Children are usually seen yearly during this time for a craniofacial team evaluation, but parents can contact their team to arrange an earlier appointment if concerns arise.
- Paying attention to their child's early school performance, particularly reading skills. They can talk with the school or team psychologist about having the child tested to rule out learning problems. The sooner a diagnosis is made, the sooner intervention can begin. Early intervention can help prevent the development of emotional or behavioral problems.
- Providing opportunities for their child to socialize and develop positive peer relationships and interests (for example, sports and other extracurricular activities).
- Offering coaching if their child is shy. This includes role playing conversations and allowing time to warm up in new situations. Children who are shy can join an activity or group to help build friendships.
- Teaching their child good social skills such as making eye contact when talking with others, ways to start and maintain a conversation with a new peer, and how to be a good listener.
- Resisting the urge to overprotect their child. Parenting is like flying a kite— if parents hold their child too closely all the time, he or she won't learn how to fly.
- Educating siblings about CLP. Parents can talk with their other children to understand their concerns and questions and to give them opportunities to have individual attention.
- Continuing to teach their child about CLP. The child should have a brief explanation to use when others ask about a difference ("I was born with a cleft or a split in my lip. I had surgery to fix it, and now I have this scar, but it doesn't hurt. Hey, I just got this new game, would you like to play?"). This can help their child feel in control of the situation and less anxious.

- Preparing their child for medical procedures. Some children do better with more information; some do better with less. Most children's hospitals have child life specialists who help children learn about where they will be and what will happen when they come to the hospital. Siblings often have worries about their brother's or sister's surgery and can benefit from these services as well.
- Helping their child develop a positive body image by modeling such an image themselves. For example, parents should not talk negatively about their own or another person's appearance in the presence of their child. Children's feelings need to be validated. Parents can remind their child that we are all unhappy about some aspect of our own appearance. Children can be encouraged to focus on what their body can do as opposed to how it looks and to think about positive aspects of their appearance. Parents can compliment their child on his or her abilities, talents, and other characteristics, as well as appearance.
- Teasing and bullying are issues that can affect every child, not only children with CLP. All children should be educated about how to respond if they are teased or bullied (for example, the child can tell an adult, respond neutrally, and/or walk away).

Adolescence and Beyond

As children enter adolescence, they look to become more independent from their family. Relationships with peers take on increasing importance and can influence interests and activities. Although peers become more important, many adolescents with CLP report feeling close with their families and continue to receive a lot of support from family members. Teenagers will begin to consider career interests and educational plans beyond high school.

Adolescence is a time when most if not all people become more aware of their appearance and attractiveness, particularly as interest in dating increases. Teenagers are commonly self-conscious about their appearance, in part because of changes related to puberty and physical growth. Research indicates that most adolescents with CLP have good self-concepts, although the risk for low self-concept can be a concern, particularly with regard to popularity and appearance. Adolescents with appearance and/or speech differences can be at risk for teasing and bullying; being singled out for having a different appearance can be particularly distressing for teenagers.

Because adolescence is the time when physical maturity is achieved, it is a time when additional surgical procedures can be discussed. Teenagers can feel conflicted about having more surgery. They worry about missing school, activities, and time with friends. Sometimes teenagers want to have surgery to improve their appearance, but they may also be fearful of attention from peers about changes in their appearance after surgery. Parents can be inclined to encourage their teenager to have surgery now, because they can understand the short- and long-term risks and benefits more clearly. Practical concerns, such as having surgery while insurance coverage is still available, factor into decisions about surgery.

Research about psychological adjustment in adults with CLP is fairly limited; most studies of adults with CLP were conducted decades ago and found that they were less likely to marry and more likely to have more social and employment problems. However, these findings likely have little relevance for today's youth, given the dramatic changes that have occurred in surgical care and in the types of services and interventions that are offered to children with CLP.

By the time a cleft-affected child enters young adulthood, he or she will probably graduate from team care, because most medical treatments will have been completed. Parents and their adolescent or older child often reflect on their experience over the years and the positive and negative effects. Parents commonly have questions about what happens at this stage if their child develops a cleft-related concern (for example, speech or dental problems) or if their child decides to pursue additional surgery. The child may have questions about family planning and whether his or her own children will have CLP. For some young adults, appearance and social concerns persist; depression and anxiety can develop, particularly for those who are dissatisfied with their appearance or have struggled with self-esteem and social relationships.

What Parents Can Do to Promote Resilience

Parents can help their adolescent or young adult child develop resilience in many ways, including:
- Continuing to encourage participation in activities to foster social relationships.
- Monitoring their child's academic performance and consider options for college or vocational training.
- Encouraging their child to participate in decision-making about their health care and procedures. Parents can talk with their child about the pros and cons of having or delaying surgery. The child can bring a list of questions to team appointments and talk with team members directly (rather than having parents take the lead). Parents should educate their child about his or her medical and surgical histories and schedule a consult with the team geneticist to discuss their child's risk of having a child with CLP.

- Continuing to model healthy body image behaviors and attitudes about appearance to show that they remember and understand how important appearance can seem at this time in their child's life. Children should be taught to think critically about media images of appearance ideals and encouraged to engage in discussions about qualities that make people attractive beyond physical appearance such as humor, confidence, and kindness.
- Talking with their child about his or her thoughts and perspectives and encouraging consideration of the benefits and positive aspects of having CLP.
- Encouraging their child to talk with a psychologist if he or she has appearance or social concerns or is struggling with anxiety or depression. Treatments such as cognitive behavioral therapy can improve body image and social skills and decrease anxiety and depression.

CONCLUSION

Raising a child with CLP can present challenges for parents but also opportunities to teach skills and lessons that contribute to well-being over time. The ultimate goal of team care is to support the well-being and quality of life of children with CLP and of their families. Parents and craniofacial team mental health specialists can work together to minimize the potential for psychosocial problems by being aware of risks and taking steps to identify and address them.

10

Educating the Child With Cleft Lip and Palate

Donna Cutler-Landsman

KEY POINTS

- Early intervention is particularly helpful in decreasing the severity of language and literacy deficits in cleft-affected children.

- It is crucial for school personnel to fully understand and address the special needs of this group of children.

- Schools need to address not only educational issues for cleft-affected children, but also bullying and self-esteem concerns.

- Cleft-affected children diagnosed with 22q11.2 deletion syndrome, also known as velocardiofacial or DiGeorge syndrome, have more intensive educational challenges.

Shepherding children through the educational processes and stages can be a daunting task for most parents. For families with children who have unique learning and/or medical needs, it can be a particularly challenging journey. Parents often find themselves in the position of having to balance a positive working relationship with the school with their need to advocate for more specialized services for their child. In today's world of budget cuts and dwindling resources, parents must take an active role in the educational process and understand their child's rights and the school's responsibility to ensure that their child receives an appropriate education.

The task of educating a child with cleft lip and palate needs to be a collaborative effort among medical professionals, therapists, educators, and family. All parties need to work cooperatively to craft carefully orchestrated programs that address all aspects of child development. Any area that is neglected can quickly derail progress and can have lasting detrimental effects. Therefore working as a team is imperative to ensure the best possible educational outcome for these students.

Although most cleft-affected children require speech and language therapy, their educational needs can vary significantly. Some need minimal school-based therapy or classroom interventions, whereas others have complex learning needs requiring specialized, individual programs throughout their school years. Each child is unique, and frequent assessment and data collection are essential to provide an appropriately tailored program. Research indicates that early intervention, preferably during preschool, kindergarten, and early elementary school, is particularly helpful in decreasing the severity of language and literacy deficits. Therefore early initiation of speech and language therapy is prudent.

Succeeding in school involves much more than the ability to speak clearly. Issues such as receptive and expressive language skills, hearing, higher-order thinking skills, and the use of pragmatic language in everyday life affect a student's ability to learn and eventually live independently. A student's school-based therapy program must take into account all of the variables that impede learning and success in the classroom. This includes many broader aspects of speech and language such as the following:

- The ability to listen and understand multistep directions
- The skills to communicate with classmates and make friends
- The ability and confidence to present and explain learned material to others
- The cognitive capability to understand the nuances of language
- The ability to learn more technical vocabulary in content area classes

To craft a comprehensive and integrated program, school personnel need to fully understand the needs of the child in all of these domains. An interdisciplinary team approach involving medical personnel, therapists, early learning special educators, and families is required to fully understand and execute a thorough educational plan.

Early and aggressive speech and language therapy during the formative years provides the child with the best opportunity to enter kindergarten with optimal speech and language skills. For most children born with a cleft condition, a realistic goal should be normal speech and language usage by the time they are of school age.

EARLY INTERVENTION PROGRAMS THROUGH THE SPECIAL EDUCATION SYSTEM

Once it becomes apparent that a child has a lip or palate irregularity, parents can contact the school system to see if it offers an early intervention program to provide speech and language therapy and other services. Doctors and their staff can be contacted to help facilitate the referral. In the United States, children with disabilities or developmental delays are entitled to early intervention services under a federal law known as the *Individuals With Disabilities Education Act,* Part C. This entitlement begins when the child is born. These services are called Birth to Three Programs and are often funded by Part C of the Individuals With Disabilities Education Act. Although these programs differ slightly from state to state, the guiding principles are summarized as follows:

- Children's optimal development depends on their being viewed first as children and second as children with a problem or disability.
- Children's greatest resource is their family.
- Parents are partners in any activity that serves their children.
- Just as children are best supported within the context of family, the family is best supported within the context of the community.
- Professionals are most effective when they can work as a team member with parents and others.
- Collaboration is the best way to provide comprehensive services.
- Early intervention enhances the development of children.

Although, at first, it may be difficult for parents to adjust to the realization that their child has special needs, there are numerous reasons to be optimistic about long-term results. Today, many services are available, and educational outcomes are very positive for children who receive the necessary intervention services. Parents should be assured that procedural safeguards are in place to protect their right to confidentiality, and that regulations exist that will allow families to be an integral part of the educational planning process. Parents also have the right to refuse services or to file a complaint if they think their child's needs are not being addressed adequately. Families are allowed to bring in outside experts or advocates, such as private therapists, doctors, special education experts, and consultants, to assist in the school planning process.

Special Education Process

Initial referrals for special education services should be made through the state Department of Health and Human Services. Families can find the contact number for their agency online, through the phone directory, or by asking their medical providers. They should ask for the Birth to Three Program intake coordinator. Parents should also contact their local school system for assistance in this process. After the initial referral is made, an eligibility process will follow to determine if the child meets the criteria for services. In most states, the child must have a significant delay to be eligible for assistance. A formal evaluation is performed to determine whether the child qualifies for an early intervention program. This process will include testing, interviews, and observations.

Testing Considerations for Very Young Children

Several tests are available for therapists to use to determine educational eligibility for speech and language services. The American Speech and Hearing Association website has information on several of these assessments. Although the primary focus of early intervention therapy for students with cleft palate is usually articulation, educational evaluations should also assess underlying language deficits. Examples of suggested instruments that focus on language development are the following:

- *The Communication and Symbolic Behavior Scales Development Profile* (ages 8 to 24 months): This assessment indicates deficits in verbal and social interaction skills.
- *The Symbolic Play Test* (ages 1-3 years): This test helps to identify the early skills needed for language development and the child's early concept formation and ability to symbolize.
- *Reynell Developmental Language Scales* (ages 1 to 6 years): This assessment identifies delays in verbal comprehension and expressive language skills.

After assessments confirm that a child is eligible for services, a plan should be developed quickly (often within 30 days) to optimize outcomes. This plan, referred to as an *Individual Family Service Plan,* outlines the special supports and services that will be provided. For children from birth to 3 years of age, the program focuses on the family, and services are provided in the young child's natural environment, usually the home. The special education program targets the entire family and centers on how those closest to the child can support the learning and developmental goals. Individual service plans include services from education resources, health and social services agencies, and informal networks and resources. The plan includes the following information:

- The child's present level of performance across all developmental domains, including vision, hearing, and health
- A statement of goals
- Support services that will be provided to meet the goals
- The date services will begin
- The name of the person who will be coordinating the services

For children with cleft lip and palate, services usually focus on language acquisition and development of intelligible speech. For some infants and toddlers who display more complex needs, interventions can include occupational and physical therapy and cognitive remediation programs.

Preschool Programs

After the child is 3 years of age, special education services shift from family-based interventions to a program centered on the child. At this juncture, a transition plan is written to usually move services from the home environment to a formal preschool setting. Some districts, however, choose to have therapists provide services on an itinerant basis in the child's home or a daycare setting. Regardless of the setting, the plan changes from an individual family service plan to an *individual education plan* (IEP) and targets academic achievement and functional performance.

The IEP must be reviewed at least annually to determine whether goals are being met. Parents can request a more frequent review if it is warranted by the situation. An extended school year can also be requested that will allow services to continue over the summer months. This can be especially important for children with a cleft palate who need uninterrupted speech therapy after or before repair surgeries. Parents are encouraged to ask professionals working with their child to provide written documentation that can be presented at IEP meetings, indicating the frequency of speech therapy sessions recommended by medical personnel. This type of collaboration between medical staff and the school system is extremely helpful in securing necessary services.

Children with articulation and language difficulties often present special challenges both at home and at school. The inability to verbally express needs in an understandable manner can be frustrating for the child and teacher/caregiver. In addition, difficulty being understood can lead to limited language use by the child when the attempts to use more complicated language are not reinforced by the listener. The classroom teacher and parents can use several approaches to help manage these issues and improve speech and language development. The following suggestions can be helpful for parents and teachers:

- Self-talk can be used, in which adults describe what they are doing and label items in the environment.
- Parallel talk is useful and involves describing what the child is doing.
- Adults can embellish the child's speech, restating and enhancing it by adding additional details.
- Adults can rephrase or restate what the child says to add more colorful language and improve vocabulary.
- Practice techniques such as dialogic reading can enhance oral language skills (*http://www.readingrockets.org/article/400/Whitehurst*).

- Gestures or symbols can help the child communicate until he or she achieves intelligible speech. Picture boards, computers, and photographs can be helpful.
- Adults can initiate a behavior modification program to reward appropriate behavior if outbursts or tantrums are a problem.
- Adults can encourage peer interaction in a group setting and monitor and facilitate social interchanges.

SCHOOL-BASED PROGRAMS FOR CHILDREN WITH CLEFT LIP AND PALATE

As a child enters a public school program in kindergarten, a new IEP will be drafted to describe the services that will be offered, including speech and language therapy, academic support, and related services such as occupational and/or physical therapy. Having a cleft palate and/or speech needs does not automatically qualify a child for special education services under the Individuals With Disabilities Education Act. The IEP team must determine that the level of speech and language impairment is sufficient to affect the child's ability to benefit from a free and appropriate education. The team will look at such things as the child's ability to be understood by the teacher and other students; the extent to which the language impairment interferes with the child's ability to read, write, and communicate; the impact that the speech difficulty has on social interactions; and the child's willingness to orally participate in classroom activities. Many children with minor speech differences do not receive formalized services through the public school system. Instead, a home exercise program may be designed, allowing the child to practice targeted speech skills at home. Sometimes a wait-and-see approach is suggested for children who have minor articulation issues that do not seem to cause much difficulty academically. This is done because speech can develop as the children matures, making formalized speech and language therapy unnecessary. As mentioned previously, it is quite helpful if the medical team treating the child writes a letter outlining the suggested number of therapy sessions for the child's condition to help secure school services.

Speech and Language Testing for School-Age Children

Therapists need to consider issues in addition to articulation when testing children for speech and language services in school. Although some children with cleft lip and palate seem to progress well developmentally, others have underlying language deficits that will significantly affect their academic success. Some educators erroneously assume that the delay in language is caused only by physical issues associated with the palate, and that the problem will resolve after surgical intervention, when speech articulation improves. On the contrary, some children with irregularities (such as those with 22q11.2 deletion syndrome) have additional neurocognitive deficits that result in lifelong struggles with pragmatic language and abstract, higher-level thinking concepts. After having palate surgery and speech therapy to correct severe hypernasality and articulation errors early in life, most children with 22q11.2 deletion syndrome develop near-normal speaking capabilities and meet their articulation IEP goals. Some IEP teams have erroneously dismissed these children from speech and language services, even though receptive and expressive language deficits are routinely associated with this syndrome and affect these students throughout their lifetimes.

Schools frequently review only the average quotient score on assessments and fail to recognize and consider the child's strengths and weaknesses on subtests. Very often, children with significant difficulties are found ineligible for services, because high performance on one test section skews the result. To more carefully analyze a child's need for therapy services, it is recommended that testing extend beyond basic speech skills and include assessments of problem-solving and higher-order thinking ability. Suggested language-based assessments include the following:

- Comprehensive Assessment of Spoken Language (ages 3 to 22 years)
- Test of Problem Solving 3 (elementary [ages 6 to 12 years] and adolescent [ages 12 to 17 years] versions are available)
- Test of Pragmatic Language (ages 6 to 19 years)
- Token Test (ages 3 to 13 years)

Pullout Services in Schools

Speech therapy services in school can be delivered in many different approaches, including one-on-one or small group pullout interventions or classroom-based services. The research is mixed as to whether one approach produces more positive outcomes than another. Although public schools most commonly use the pullout service delivery model, there is interest in assessing whether this modality is the most desirable for all children. A better approach would be to individualize services according to the needs of the child.

Speech therapy using a pullout approach may be very appropriate when the goals are articulation based. A small group or individualized setting can offer unique advantages for treatment, especially when children are first learning to use specific skills. This quieter, targeted setting allows the therapist and the child to rehearse skills unrelated to the classroom curriculum. Additional home practice exercises and a reinforcement program in the classroom for intelligible speech can be incorporated and may be all that is needed.

However, in many cases, a more intensive program is indicated. Children with cleft lip and palate need to be tested extensively for language deficits, and the testing should be repeated, at least several years after a surgical intervention. Furthermore, intervention may need to be much more intensive and frequent. Some evidence shows that language-based intervention in the school is most successful when it is delivered on a daily basis, sustains the child's attention, and involves corrective feedback and positive reinforcement. Additionally, therapy that incorporates concepts that are currently relevant in the classroom helps the child understand classroom discussions and improve literacy skills. This approach will require that speech and language pathologists work closely with regular and special education staff to coordinate services and modify classroom curricula. The regular education teacher (who typically has the most contact with the child) should be informed about the therapy goals and given specific strategies for facilitating improvement. Too often, there is a disconnection between the classroom setting and the therapy room.

Scheduling conflicts can make this collaborative approach difficult for schools to use. Creative problem-solving, such as grouping students with similar needs in one classroom, can make this a viable delivery model. Speech and language pathologists who specialize in particular grade levels (lower versus upper elementary, for example) become more intimately familiar with the curriculum and the teaching styles of the staff in the building. Planning curriculum modifications can be quite time consuming. Speech and language pathologists who work with fewer teachers can more easily rewrite tests to modify the complexity of language, prepare study guides, and highlight textbooks to identify main ideas. Collaborative release times for interventions can be specifically written into the IEP to facilitate a team approach. IEPs are most effective when staff is given the needed support to plan, develop materials, and work together.

SPECIAL EDUCATIONAL CONSIDERATIONS

22q11.2 Deletion Syndrome

Children with 22q11.2 deletion syndrome (also known as velocardiofacial or DiGeorge syndrome) may have a cleft palate as well as other medical conditions that are the result of the genetic syndrome. They have complex learning needs and require more than speech and language therapy alone. This syndrome affects approximately 1 in 2000 to 4000 students. These children have the following additional educational concerns:

- Developmental delay occurs, especially in the emergence of language.
- Cognition is impaired. IQ is lower than expected (below 70 in 30% of children).

- A large discrepancy exists between verbal and performance abilities. Many children have a verbal IQ significantly higher than their performance IQ, which may be evidence of a nonverbal learning disability.
- Approximately 90% of children present with learning difficulties that require specialized interventions from school personnel. Most have severe math impairment and difficulty with reading comprehension.
- Approximately 20% of these children have autism or autistic spectrum disorder. Many more demonstrate social skill deficits.
- Behavior difficulties (usually attention issues) occur, but obsessive behaviors are common.
- At least 60% of affected students develop a psychiatric disorder. Schizophrenia is detected in 25% of adults.
- Muscle tone is low, and occupational or physical therapy is needed.
- Visual/spatial deficits interfere with visual discrimination, visual memory, and form constancy.
- Life skills acquisition is typically lower than expected.

School personnel are strongly encouraged to familiarize themselves with this highly unrecognized but relatively common syndrome. Many children go undetected for years before the genetic syndrome is identified as the underlying cause of the child's academic and medical challenges.

Management of Psychological Problems

Bullying and self-esteem are concerns for cleft-affected children, just as they are for children with other disabilities. Schools must actively work to ensure that students feel accepted, comfortable, and valued. Psychological problems such as anxiety and depression are more prevalent in children with cleft lip and palate. Schools need to actively address these issues through student support groups or in the IEP. Students with 22q11.2 deletion syndrome are particularly vulnerable to developing psychological problems.

Schools can do a great deal to help foster a climate of acceptance among students. School-wide antibullying programs, social skills groups, and counseling services can help to address the psychosocial issues in these children. Students should be screened for psychological issues associated with their speech and language, and goals should be added to the IEP to address areas of concern. Special care is required as these students enter adolescence, which is a time when self-image and friendships become more of an issue. Some researchers have indicated that as children with cleft lip and palate mature, they become more dissatisfied with their appearance. By this age, students may have been dismissed from speech therapy services in the public schools. Parents, however, can contact the school for support if they think their child is in need of supportive services.

CONCLUSION

Effective school programming is possible for students with cleft lip and palate. The approach must be multidisciplinary and collaborative. Medical personnel and parents play key roles in assisting school personnel in understanding how to best serve these students. Carefully tailored education plans should address not only articulation, but also language, academic, social, and emotional needs. All aspects of development need to be considered when the need for special education intervention is assessed. As students mature, they need to be followed to actively address self-esteem, academic, social, and communication issues that can develop. Working together, with proactive supports, will hopefully produce a bright and productive future for this group of students.

11

The Role of the Social Worker on the Cleft Team

Cassandra L. Aspinall

KEY POINTS

- This chapter helps parents of cleft-affected children and other family members understand the role of social workers. One goal is to encourage the family to receive the beneficial advocacy that social workers provide.

- Social workers are highly qualified experts in social issues. They can help families with challenges they have with others, including people at work and insurance providers.

- The social worker's role is to help the family understand current complex medical plans and treatments.

- Language and cultural barriers can create fear, confusion, and apprehension about social workers, particularly for families from diverse ethnic backgrounds. Social workers are obligated to assist families as they meet these obstacles.

- Social workers have many responsibilities, including identifying extra support and resources needed by the patient and family, communicating the family's needs and obstacles with the health care team, and helping the family identify their strengths in caring for their child.

When a family learns of their child's craniofacial diagnosis prenatally or after birth, each family member will need to make adjustments. Every family has unique needs that need to be considered by the cleft or craniofacial team as it develops a treatment plan for the child. The team becomes acquainted with the family and potential care issues during the child's full medical evaluation. As reviewed in Chapter 1, each member of the cleft or craniofacial team serves a different role in the child's treatment. The social worker is a member of the team who helps to identify the challenges that the patient, family, and cleft team may face in providing optimal patient care. Further, the social worker assists the patient, family, and team members in overcoming these obstacles.

For example, the medical terminology associated with the child's condition may be new to the family. Additionally, the specific needs of every family will be new to the health care team. The social worker can help to explain these medical terms and identify the family's needs.

The training of a social worker is focused on learning assessment and intervention tools that help the team understand the patient and family. These professionals have a breadth of training and knowledge on human behavior and interaction throughout development. They are also trained in group dynamics and societal structures focused on accessing the following supplementary resources:
- Financial and employment support
- Mental health and counseling referrals
- Complementary therapies (for example, speech-language therapy)
- Legal and insurance issues
- Transportation
- Education

Social workers identify factors that might interfere with a patient's care plan. They are trained to meet with families to determine the language, cultural, spiritual, and other critical family values that need to be considered in the plan of care. These factors are then communicated to the rest of the health care team for consideration as they develop a treatment plan.

The social worker's primary ethical obligation is to the child. This is true of each member of the health care team. The parent or guardian is the child's best advocate.

A child with extra medical needs often requires more resources. The emotional stress can be hard to cope with, especially if other issues in the family are already causing stress. Parents with a smaller support network (for example, other family members or members of their place of worship) may have more stress while caring for a child with a cleft lip and/or palate. An extended social network can help tremendously. The social worker can provide the family with important tips and guidance as the child progresses through treatment.

A SOCIAL WORKER'S TOOLS: THE BASIC BIOPSYCHOSOCIAL ASSESSMENT

A social worker is uniquely trained to help patients and families cope with the stress of the child's diagnosis. The social worker determines the needs of the patient and family through basic assessments across the patient's lifespan. This assessment is known as a *biopsychosocial assessment* and is repeated at specific times throughout a child's treatment to make sure that new information is taken into consideration. The following factors will be assessed by the social worker:
- Emotional reactions to news of the diagnosis
- Communication with family and friends to determine who can be counted on to help
- A review of the family's medical resources
  - Who are the family's doctor and the baby's doctor?
  - Who are the dentist and the orthodontist?
  - What are the family's insurance issues?
- The family's current financial situation
  - What is the employment status of the caregivers?
  - Time away from work. Families may be eligible for income through the *Family and Medical Leave Act* (FMLA).
  - State support. Families may be eligible for support through the Temporary Aid to Needy Families program, the Special Supplemental Nutrition for Women, Infants and Children program, and supplemental security income.
  - What are the family's concerns about household bills and food?
- Housing
  - Is the family housing shared or temporary?
  - How long has the family lived at the current location?
  - Do the parents pay mortgage or rent?
- Transportation
  - Is the family vehicle shared?
  - The family's ability to attend appointments. (Will the vehicle be available? What is the cost of travel?)
- Family constellation
  - Where do family members live—in the house or elsewhere?

- Are siblings available to provide care? Do they require their own care from the parents?
- Who are the friends and/or extended family members who provide child care or care for other dependent relatives or individuals?
- Informal community support
  - Friends of the family
  - The family's place of worship
  - The availability of daycare support
- Stressful situations in the house before the child's medical situation was diagnosed
  - Drug or alcohol abuse issues
  - Mental health treatment
  - Domestic violence and/or other safety concerns
  - Medical health issues
- Previous experience with this diagnosis or other medical conditions and time in hospitals or other treatment environments

Once a baseline assessment is completed, the social worker will find the resources needed to reduce existing problems and prevent new ones. Potential issues such as unemployment, homelessness, poverty, domestic violence, mental illness, and substance abuse are difficult to cope with and add increased stress to the families of cleft-affected children.

TIMELINE OF ASSESSMENTS

Prenatal Assessments

The diagnosis of a cleft lip and/or palate is often made during a prenatal ultrasound examination. This technology is not exact; therefore, physicians will usually discuss the possibility that the child will have this condition. The social worker will talk with the parents after the initial prenatal workup to understand their emotional state, which will greatly influence how the family will cope with the information about their child.

The social worker has several important things to review at this time, including the medical facts related to the care of the newborn and the care that the child will need as he or she matures. The social worker will discuss these needs with the parents, incorporating other topics into the conversations, including the parents' emotional reaction to the diagnosis, the effect of the cleft on the newborn's feeding, and the child's potential speech issues. Facial clefts can be accompanied by other conditions; the social worker will discuss these possibilities with the parents. Social workers encourage parents to connect with other parents of children with cleft-related differences by providing information and referrals to support networks.

Parents who are expecting a cleft-affected child can have intense feelings of guilt after learning of their child's condition; family members sometimes blame the pregnant mother. The physician will give parents medical information about how clefts occur in an effort to dispel misconceptions. The social worker on the team will focus on what the family thinks caused the cleft. Such beliefs are often very deeply held and are not always swayed by medical facts, even if the cause is genetic. By offering parents the opportunity to talk about how they are coping with all of this new information, the social worker can greatly help to ease their guilt.

Expecting parents appreciate the chance to talk about how their resources and time planning may have to be adjusted based on the arrival of their baby. Examples of resources that are explored by social workers include health insurance (medical and dental), employment-related concerns (short-term and long-term medical absence), daycare, and the effect on siblings.

Social workers will ask parents if and with whom they have discussed the diagnosis. Many parents worry about the reaction of others. A social worker can help to prepare parents for the many different responses they might receive when they tell others about their child's condition. On the other hand, if they are not sure how to initiate this dialogue, the social worker will provide advice about how to begin.

Many parents will have intense emotional suffering and grief after they are told that their child may have a facial difference. They worry that their child will suffer from the difference even though it is not a life-threatening condition. The social worker will discuss postpartum depression with the mother to make sure that she has the proper support after the birth of her child. The intensity of these feelings can be reduced if the parent processes these strong emotions in counseling, with close friends or support networks, and with his or her partner. Keeping such feelings suppressed can lead to problems with depression and physical symptoms such as sleeplessness and lack of appetite. These concerns warrant a referral for further assessment and treatment.

The social worker will speak openly with parents about the child's psychological and social health. The parent's fears will be discussed, and they will be given specific advice about what should or should not be a concern. Social workers treat all cases based on the family's and patient's unique needs. For example, in some families, the parent also has a cleft. This parent's concerns may be different from those of parents who do not have a cleft. The social worker might discuss concepts of parental resilience to cope with unpredicted childhood adversity such as illness and traumatic accidents. Parents appreciate the reminder that they will rise to the occasion to protect and help their child in any circumstance.

The social worker might ask some of the following questions at the prenatal appointment:

- Do you feel prepared for the delivery, and do you have enough emotional and physical support?
- As a family, do you worry about the immediate financial impact related to missing work, having to travel, or paying insurance expenses?
- Have you thought through how to introduce your baby to family, friends, and the public?
- Are you having symptoms of depression, such as sleeplessness and lack of appetite?

Newborn Assessments

The newborn meeting with the social worker and the prenatal meeting with the social worker share many similarities. Although facial clefts often can be diagnosed in utero through ultrasound technology, this is not always true. The cleft is not always detected before birth. Additionally, a parent whose child has a cleft palate without a cleft lip will most likely learn of this difference at the delivery. No matter what happened before the child's birth, the social worker will explain to the parents how their child will be cared for immediately after birth.

Parents who are included in the care of their child at delivery and kept informed about their child's condition will often report having less fear about their child's well-being. Parents who are separated from their cleft-affected newborn sometimes struggle to trust medical providers at this very emotional time. They might worry about their own abilities to parent a child with this condition. At the newborn visit, the parents will share their experience at the time of delivery. This discussion is essential for establishing a strong foundation between the cleft or craniofacial team and the family.

At the newborn assessment, the social worker meets with the parents and infant to discuss the basic history of the family and several other important factors. For example, the social worker may ask about the immediate family's reaction to the baby's appearance and about the family's state of mind and how they are coping. Although this discussion may make the family uncomfortable, it is important for the family to know that guilt and fear are typical emotions.

For a child with a cleft palate who is not able to breast-feed, the physician and nursing staff will often be in charge of reviewing feeding mechanics. The process of pumping breast milk and using specialized bottles is often overwhelming for mothers and their families. Adding to this stress is the mother's sense of loss from not being able to breast-feed. Many parents are concerned whether the insurance company will pay for equipment such as specialized bottles and breast pumps. Social workers can help to relieve some of the emotional reactions to the parents' feeding concerns by working with insurance companies to ensure payment for noncontracted but medically necessary equipment.

At the newborn appointment, a social worker can begin to work with the parents to coordinate home and work schedules according to their baby's needs. Some families may have already completed FMLA paperwork to explain the mother's absence from work because of her pregnancy. After the child is born, the family may need help filling out new forms to document the expected absences of the mother and the father from their workplaces. FMLA protection does not guarantee payment beyond what an individual may have from traditional sick leave, vacation, or paid time off. However, this documentation can protect an employee from losing a job or promotion based on concerns about absences. Such paperwork can explain that the parent will not only need to be away from work for blocks of time (for example, for the child's surgery), but also for intermittent absences for therapy visits (for example, speech-language therapy and feedings) and frequent medical visits beyond the expected well-child checks at the pediatrician's office.

Working with other team specialists helps the family to access early intervention services (for example, through an individulalized family service plan) or financial support through supplemental security income. These resources help to support children and families with the costs of specialized medical treatments. To determine the needs of the family, the social worker will ask questions such as the following:
- Does your family have enough of the basic resources to provide the day-to-day and specialty care your baby needs, including food, shelter, safety, and support?
- Do you need referrals to supplement your resources (for example, a public health nurse consult in the community, food bank, or other help)?
- Do you need documentation regarding any change in your work plan and/or return to work after meeting your baby and finalizing the newborn care plan?
- If you feel overwhelmed, do you have someone close to home to talk to?
- Do you understand the next steps in your baby's care plan and know who to contact if you have questions?

Surgical Preparation Assessments

Most infants with clefts require surgery. Social workers will work with the other health care team members and the parents so that they know that their child's needs are being met by the team. The team will also make sure that the parents understand the medical and surgical treatment plan. The more a parent understands about the process, the less they will fear for their child's well-being. Social workers will understand the parents' fears concerning the cost of the treatment and will help the family understand what to expect financially. The social worker will ask the following questions before surgery to determine whether the family is prepared for the upcoming financial obligations:

- Do you have enough money for the extra food and travel (with lodging) that may be needed around the time of the child's surgery and recovery?
- Will you be able to miss work without a problem?
- How much of your time away from work will affect your family's budget?
- Do you have family and/or friends who can help?
- Would you like help in applying for supplemental funding sources if needed?
- Are both parents available to help with the hospitalization and discharge care?
- Do any of the adults who will be involved in the care of the child (parents included) have mental health or other issues, such as anxiety or substance abuse, that could be worsened by being in a hospital setting?
- Are you concerned about safety issues such as domestic violence that might affect your safety or the safety of your child after discharge from the hospital?
- Have you thought about your reaction to the dramatic change in your child's appearance?

As the child get older, the social worker can discuss expectations and expected benefits from surgery. These conversations will help the social worker to ensure that negative experiences are not repeated.

Surgical Decision-Making Assessments

Some surgical procedures are focused on improving a vital physical function, whereas others are meant to improve the quality of a patient's life. The initial operations to close clefts of the lip and palate, alveolar bone graft surgery (see Chapter 29), nasal surgery to improve breathing, midfacial/jaw surgery, and placement of ear tubes are a few examples of operations performed primarily to improve function. Revision procedures that further correct deformities of the lip and nose are designed to benefit the patient's quality of life by improving appearance.

Making surgical decisions can be difficult for parents and patients alike. They must determine whether the benefits of an operation to improve function or appearance outweigh potential risks. Social workers can participate in conversations between team members and the family to facilitate the decision-making process. Social workers can also help to determine the timing of surgery so that the practical needs of the patient and family are best met. In many cases, the patient is verbal and can take part in the decision-making process. Sometimes, the parents' and the child's opinions differ. The team will work with the family and consider all members involved. The social worker might ask parents some of the following questions before surgery:

- How often is your child's facial difference noticed by others?
- Is the attention expressed as questions or curiosity? Are others staring? Are hurtful comments made? Do you notice whispering?
- When others notice your child's facial differences, does this disrupt your child's day?
- Have you noticed that your attention to this problem is more intense than that of your child?
- What are the disadvantages of waiting to do the surgery?
- What are the advantages of waiting to do the surgery?

Elementary School Assessments

As the child enters the elementary school age (approximately 5 to 11 years of age), a social worker will continue to meet with the family. The same basic assessment will be updated, because families change, along with their resources and thoughts about medical care. Important questions will be asked about the child's school experience. These questions are often centered on peer interaction and potential learning issues that may have developed. At this age, a child may need to be assessed by the school, the team speech-language pathologist, and a psychologist to obtain recommendations for an individualized educational plan (see Chapter 10). Some children can have signs of mental health problems such as anxiety or depression. Alternatively, as children become more settled in school and peer communities, they often develop positive coping strategies that the social worker should acknowledge and encourage.

Despite the challenges of having a visible difference that requires medical treatment, cleft-affected children can develop emotional strength because of their condition. At this age, meeting children with the same condition can be very helpful. Social workers can recommend numerous groups and summer camps across the country that will help to connect children with others who have related conditions. Social workers are trained to consider this broad spectrum of factors in the life of the child and family, while being alert to detect risk factors that can be addressed proactively, if needed. The social worker may ask the child the following questions:

- At school, are you asked questions about your appearance or speech differences?
- How do you handle these questions? Do these questions make you uncomfortable?
- Are the questions being asked in a way that is respectful and genuinely curious?
- Do you feel that others are teasing or bullying you? (It is the *child's* definition of bullying that matters when deciding whether help is needed.)

Additional questions for the parents include:

- Does the school have a protocol for dealing with bullying?
- Do you think that the school is giving your child the proper educational support for his or her learning disabilities?
- Do your child's speech or hearing problems affect his or her participation in academic and/or social settings? Are these issues being addressed?

Middle and High School Assessments

When the child is 12 to 18 years of age, the social worker's focus shifts to the emerging identity of the patient within the family and in relation to the medical team. Children develop an understanding of their condition as they mature through adolescence and into adulthood. This emerging identity affects how the health care team moves forward. During this time, the child is assessed for surgical and orthodontic treatment. Necessary treatments are then scheduled and completed.

The social worker will develop an understanding of how the family manages the child's increasing independence during this family assessment. The social worker will want to know who is present to help the patient and whether adequate financial resources are available to complete the prescribed surgical and dental goals. Dental and orthodontic treatments are sometimes covered by insurance, but often not. The social worker will be available to discuss this and any additional stressors to help secure funding if possible.

Assessment at this stage is essential, because environmental dangers such as drugs, alcohol, and community violence can attract children, particularly if they have developed mental health issues as a result of their condition. Social workers will provide an initial screening for such issues and refer the parents and the child for additional help if indicated. Some children with a craniofacial difference do not think that their negative life experiences are related to their condition. Therefore this screening is critical.

Planning for a surgery or outpatient treatments must be done carefully with consideration of the parents' and patient's schedules. High school students have strict attendance rules at school and they must complete the core curriculum to graduate. They also have important social, employment, and athletic obligations. These need to be reconciled with the necessities of medical management to prevent delays in entering college or seeking a job. The social worker plays an important role in raising awareness of, and thus preventing, such conflicts.

As patients approach adulthood, it is important to help them understand how their condition will affect their future. The social worker will remind the team and the patient that the current treatment plan will eventually end. Social workers will facilitate conversations between the team and the patient regarding ongoing care and health issues that will need to be monitored into adulthood. Young adult patients need to be supported in this transition so that they do not feel abandoned. The social worker will ensure that the young adult and the family have appropriate referrals for ongoing care, if needed, and may review the following information with the patient, family, and health care team:

- The diagnosis and the associated medical terms
- Current medical literature about the cause of cleft lip and/or palate
- Genetic information about passing the trait from parent to child
- A treatment summary for the patient's adult doctor to streamline care. This will be developed with the health care team and will include information about the patient's reactions to medicine and anesthesia.
- Specialists the patient may need to see in the future

CONCLUSION

Social workers are available to provide assistance throughout the time that the family and patient are seen by the craniofacial team. The primary role of the social worker on the team is to help the child and family coordinate the best care possible. The social worker's main priority is to create and support an open dialogue about the patient's experience. Assessment and maintenance of communication across the lifespan of the patient are essential. Social workers are trained to understand and focus on factors beyond the family's immediate environment—the social determinants of health. These highly skilled and caring individuals are essential to the well-functioning craniofacial team. The patient will gain the greatest benefit when he or she, the family, and the health care team share the same goal: the best possible quality of life.

Part III

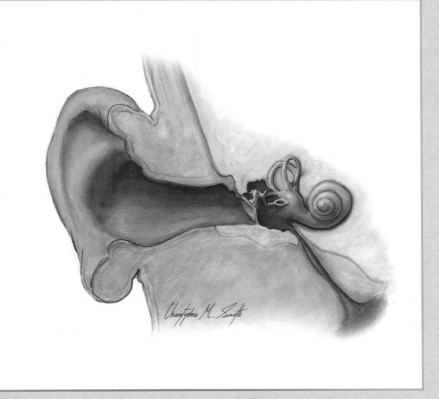

Christopher M. Smith

Cleft Palate Speech
and Hearing

12

Speech Assessment for Children With Cleft Lip and Palate

Ann W. Kummer, Adriane L. Baylis, Chelsea K. Bartley

KEY POINTS

- Children born with a cleft palate are at risk for developing a speech disorder.

- Dental abnormalities, hearing loss, and velopharyngeal insufficiency are the main causes of speech disorders in children with a cleft palate.

- Children with a cleft palate should be evaluated and treated by a speech-language pathologist as part of their care from a cleft team.

- Treatment for a speech disorder may include speech therapy, surgery, or both.

A cleft lip primarily affects the child's appearance, although speech can be affected if the cleft extends through the gum ridge (alveolus). A cleft palate affects feeding in infancy. However, the biggest concern is that a cleft palate affects the child's ability to develop normal speech. Because the palate is so important for speech, the primary goal of surgery to repair the palate *(palatoplasty)* is to provide the child with the physical ability to produce speech sounds.

Despite the lip and palate repairs, a child born with cleft lip and/or palate is at risk for having a speech disorder. Therefore evaluation by a speech-language pathologist is essential, particularly in the preschool years.

This chapter briefly describes the causes of speech disorders in children born with cleft lip and/or palate. It also informs parents of the purpose, timing, and nature of some of the procedures used in the speech evaluation. Overall, a speech assessment and follow-up are very important in the preschool years to ensure that the child's speech will eventually be normal.

CAUSES OF SPEECH DISORDERS IN CHILDREN WITH CLEFT LIP AND/OR PALATE

The main causes of speech disorders in children with cleft lip and/or palate are dental anomalies, hearing loss, and velopharyngeal insufficiency.

Dental Abnormalities

A child who has a cleft lip that extends into the alveolus can have issues with the development and position of the teeth. Missing teeth or extra teeth can be present in the area of the cleft. Some children have a malocclusion. Dental abnormalities can cause a lisp-type distortion of the teeth sounds (*s, z, sh, ch,* and *j*). They may also cause difficulty producing lip sounds (*p, b,* and *m*), teeth-lip sounds (*f* and *v*), and tongue-tip sounds (*t, d, n,* and *l*).

Hearing Loss

A child with a cleft palate has a risk of a fluctuating hearing loss because of Eustachian tube malfunction (see Chapter 14). The Eustachian tube connects the middle ear and the back of the throat *(pharynx)*. It opens during swallowing to allow fluids to drain out of the middle ear and down the back of the pharynx. It also eliminates negative air pressure within the middle ear. Children with a history of cleft palate often have poor Eustachian tube function. This is because the muscle in the soft palate that is responsible for opening the Eustachian tube does not function well. As a result, negative pressure remains and fluids build up in the middle ear. This causes frequent ear infections and temporary hearing loss. The hearing loss can affect the child's ability to develop speech skills and to learn language. To prevent middle-ear problems, *pressure-equalizing tubes* are often inserted in the eardrum at an early age. This is often done at the same time as the lip repair.

VELOPHARYNGEAL INSUFFICIENCY

The biggest concern for a child who has a cleft palate is the possibility of velopharyngeal insufficiency. This can occur in 10% to 30% of children with cleft palate, despite the palate repair.

To understand velopharyngeal insufficiency, knowledge of the relevant structures in the mouth is crucial. Fig. 12-1 shows the structures of the roof of the mouth—the hard palate and the soft palate. The soft palate is also called the *velum*.

During normal speech, air from the lungs and sound from the vocal cords, which are in the *larynx,* or voice box, travel upward in the pharynx. To produce most speech sounds, the air and sound need to be directed into the mouth and blocked from entering the nose or nasal cavity. This is done through closure of the velopharyngeal valve, which consists of the velum and the walls of the pharynx *(pharyngeal walls).*

Fig. 12-2 shows the velum resting against the back of the tongue, as occurs when a person is breathing through the nose. During inhalation, air can flow through the nose and pharynx and then down to the lungs without obstruction. Exhalation follows the same path in reverse.

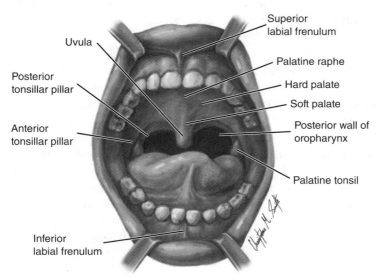

Fig. 12-1   Structures of the roof of the mouth, as seen from the front of the mouth.

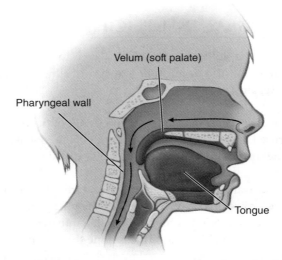

Fig. 12-2   The mouth, nasal cavity, and pharynx, as seen from the side. The velum rests against the back of the tongue while a person breathes through the nose. The *arrows* represent the inflow of air, passing through the nose and pharynx on its way to the lungs.

Fig. 12-3 shows how the velum rises against the pharyngeal walls during speech. This is velopharyngeal closure. At the same time, the pharyngeal walls at the side of the throat move inward against the soft palate. This results in a drawstring-like closure. This tight seal is needed to keep air and sound from escaping through the nose during speech and to produce all speech sounds, with the exception of *m*, *n*, and *ng*.

Fig. 12-4 shows velopharyngeal insufficiency, which is caused by a difference of the velum. In this case, the velum is too short to reach the pharyngeal wall. This condition is common in children with a history of cleft palate or submucous cleft palate (see Chapter 22).

Velopharyngeal insufficiency can cause the following speech characteristics:
- *Hypernasality,* which is the sound of too much air in the nose during speech
- Nasal emission of air during consonant production
- Weak or omitted consonants because of inadequate air pressure in the mouth
- Short utterance length resulting from the loss of air through the nose
- Altered (compensatory) speech sound production

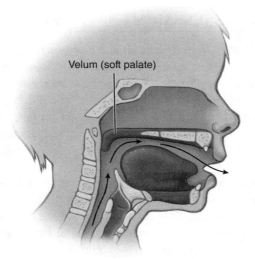

Fig. 12-3   Velopharyngeal closure. The velum rises to contact the pharyngeal walls during speech. The *arrows* show the direction of air flow from the lungs and upward through the pharynx and mouth.

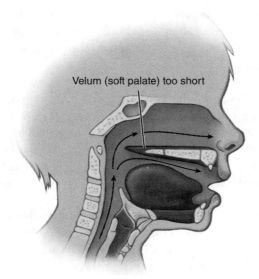

Fig. 12-4   Velopharyngeal insufficiency. The velum is too short to contact the back of the pharynx.

THE SPEECH ASSESSMENT

A child born with cleft lip and/or palate should be evaluated by a cleft or craniofacial team (see Chapter 1). Such teams are found at most major medical centers. One reason that team care is important is because the team members (who represent many different professions) specialize in the issues of children with cleft lip and/or palate. Therefore, when considering a speech assessment, a speech-language pathologist who is associated with a cleft or craniofacial team and who specializes in cleft-related speech issues should be consulted.

The craniofacial team will conduct follow-up evaluations at least yearly. At these visits, the child's general development is assessed. In the first 3 years, the speech-language pathologist is particularly concerned about the child's feeding abilities and language development. (*Language* refers to the ability to understand words and sentences that others use. It also refers to the ability to choose words and sentences when talking to others.) When the child is approximately 3 years of age, speech production and velopharyngeal function are formally assessed.

Before speech is assessed, the family is often asked to fill out a questionnaire. This is one way to determine the parents' concerns about their child's speech. It is also a way to gather information about the child's medical and development history. If the child has received any type of therapy, it is helpful to know the most recent goals and treatment approaches.

At the time of the assessment, the speech-language pathologist typically talks to the parents first to obtain additional information and to review the questionnaire as needed. Usually the child is in the room at this time so that he or she can become comfortable with the environment and the examiner. This is particularly important for children who are shy or nervous. The examiner may ask the parents if the child will cooperate better with the parents in the room or outside.

For the actual assessment, the examiner uses several methods to encourage the child to talk. This may include asking either/or questions. The examiner listens to the child's speech informally at first. Then, the examiner asks the child to name pictures, repeat certain syllables, or even repeat specific sentences to test each speech sound.

During the evaluation, the examiner looks at the child's tongue and lip placement during the production of different speech sounds. The examiner also listens to the production of each speech sound and records errors. To evaluate the velopharyngeal valve, the examiner may place a mirror under the child's nose during speech or place a straw at the tip of the child's nostril to listen for air coming through the nose. Fogging of the mirror or air heard through the straw indicate that the velopharyngeal valve may not be functioning properly.

An oral examination is another important part of the assessment. The examiner looks at the way the lips come together and examines the child's teeth and dental occlusion (the way the jaws close). The examiner also looks for a hole (*fistula*) in the repaired palate, because this may cause air to escape abnormally through the nose during speech, and for the presence of large tonsils, because they can occasionally interfere with velopharyngeal valve closure and can increase the risk of sleep apnea after surgery to correct velopharyngeal insufficiency. All observations help the examiner to determine the cause of speech errors or alterations.

In some cases, instruments are used to provide additional information about how well the velopharyngeal valve works. One commonly used instrument is the *nasometer*. This device has a microphone for the mouth and another microphone for the nose. It records sound from both microphones during speech. This information informs the examiner about a leak in the velopharyngeal valve.

RECOMMENDATIONS AFTER THE SPEECH ASSESSMENT

When the speech assessment is completed, the examiner reviews the results of testing with the parents. If speech is found to be normal, the speech-language pathologist will perform regular screening tests of speech until the child completes puberty and all treatment.

If a speech disorder is identified, the speech-language pathologist explains this to the parents and discusses treatment recommendations. These might include surgery, speech therapy, or both. If the examination shows evidence of velopharyngeal insufficiency, an additional test (*nasopharyngoscopy* or videofluoroscopy) may be recommended to determine the location and extent of the abnormal velopharyngeal opening. Velopharyngeal insufficiency always requires surgery to correct the abnormal anatomy. Speech therapy is typically necessary after the surgery.

CONCLUSION

Children with a history of cleft lip and/or palate are at risk for speech disorders. These disorders are usually caused by dental differences or velopharyngeal insufficiency. Before a child is 3 years of age, language development is the primary focus. After age 3, a formal speech assessment is necessary. The speech assessment involves a review of the parents' concerns, the child's medical and developmental history, a perceptual (listening) assessment, and an intraoral examination. Additional evaluations can be performed or recommended. The goals of the speech assessment are to identify problems as soon as possible and to develop recommendations for successful correction of all speech disorders that are diagnosed.

13

Speech Therapy for Children With Cleft Palate

Lynn Marty Grames

KEY POINTS

- o Not all children with a cleft palate require speech therapy.

- o Children with a cleft palate who need therapy can expect to have excellent speech at the conclusion of their therapy.

- o Surgery does not undo progress made in speech therapy.

- o Close communication between the family, speech-language pathologist, and cleft team is essential to obtain the best possible speech outcomes.

Early in the life of a child born with a cleft palate, many parents begin thinking about their child's speech development. They may wonder whether they will be able to understand their child's speech and what it will sound like when the child is older. Parents want to know what they can do to help their child develop normal speech.

The speech-language pathologist with the multidisciplinary cleft palate team will be able to answer many questions and provide guidance about the best plan for the child's and parents' situation. The purpose of this chapter is to offer general information about what parents should expect with their child's speech and what they can do if their child needs speech therapy. It answers often-asked questions about speech and language therapy.

Approximately 20% to 30% of children born with a cleft palate never need speech therapy and have perfectly normal speech development. The actual numbers reported vary depending on how the reporting center counted children needing speech therapy.

Approximately 70% to 80% of children born with cleft palate will have speech therapy for part of their childhood. Currently, we do not have good ways of predicting which babies will need speech therapy and which will not. For this reason, the speech-language pathologist on the cleft palate team needs to see each child on a regular basis so that speech therapy can start as soon as it is evident that speech is not developing typically. The sooner therapy starts, the sooner it ends.

Speech therapy should never be conducted simply because the child has a cleft palate. Rather, it is started because the child has a speech disorder. There is no value in starting speech therapy with babies or toddlers only because they have a cleft palate. A very young child who is one of the 20% to 30% who will develop normal speech will not benefit from this therapy.

FEEDING AND SWALLOWING THERAPY

Most babies born with a cleft palate need some early guidance and modification to feed normally. This can be provided by a nurse or speech-language pathologist who specializes in cleft palate care. Usually, no further therapy is needed. Some children with specific syndromes or medical issues or who were born prematurely may need further feeding and/or swallowing therapy. In these cases, the feeding and swallowing differences are related more to the other issues than to the cleft palate.

THE GOALS OF SPEECH THERAPY IN CHILDREN WITH CLEFT PALATE

Children who have a cleft palate, with or without a cleft lip, and no other significant medical or developmental problems should expect to develop completely normal speech. This is the goal of team care. A child should never graduate from speech therapy because he or she speaks fairly well for a child with a cleft palate or has developed speech that is as good as it can be for a child with a cleft palate. A child should graduate from speech therapy because his or her speech is normal, like that of peers.

Ideally, all children born with a cleft palate who need speech therapy will graduate from speech therapy before they begin kindergarten. This happens for many children. However, for some children this is not possible for various reasons. The next best goal is for children to graduate from speech therapy with completely normal speech by the time they begin active care with an orthodontist. This is a reasonable goal, but it requires time, diligence, and appropriate speech therapy supported by proper home programs.

Some children have other developmental or neurologic issues or a syndrome that includes a cleft palate. For these children, the possibility of needing speech therapy, the course of speech therapy, and the outcome are related to the other issue as well as the cleft palate. The cleft team's speech-language pathologist will probably be able to share information regarding expectations, given the child's particular physical and medical condition.

THE ROLE OF EARLY INTERVENTION

In a published study, children with a cleft palate who had *early intervention* were compared with children with a cleft palate who did not have early intervention. The authors found no difference in speech development between the two groups. This may occur because many speech-language pathologists have little or no training in cleft palate speech. Early intervention programs can have value for some children if the therapists are willing to collaborate with the cleft palate team. A cleft team that refers parents and their child to an early intervention program will probably be able to guide them in finding quality services and provide information and collaboration with the early intervention therapist. Some early intervention programs will offer direct, structured therapy. Other programs use a naturalistic approach, in which parents are taught to teach their child.

Parents whose child is already in an early intervention program should ask themselves these questions:
- Have I been told exactly what concerns are being addressed?
- Is the therapist explaining the therapy to me in a way that I understand?
- Do my child's communication skills seem to be getting better because of the therapy?
- Do I feel like an important part of the process?
- Is my medical team communicating with the early intervention therapist?

Parents who answer "yes" to each of these questions are typically satisfied with their child's early intervention. One or more "no" answers means that they might not be receiving the full possible benefit from the program, and it would be useful to speak with the therapist about questions and concerns.

An advantage to participation in early intervention is that the therapist and caseworker will help parents transition to the early childhood program in the local school district when the child is 3 years of age. This can reduce stress and save time in the process of preparing the child for school.

UNDERSTANDING SPEECH PROBLEMS IN CHILDREN WITH A CLEFT PALATE

Most children born with a cleft palate who need speech therapy have *articulation* disorders. These children have learned to make consonant sounds incorrectly. This disorder can develop because of the way the baby experimented with sounds while they were babbling before the cleft palate was repaired. It can occur if the baby did not hear well because of fluid in the ears or ear infections. Rarely, articulation disorders result from the shape of the child's mouth or teeth. Even more rarely, it is caused by muscle weakness *(dysarthria)* or difficulty sequencing speech muscle movements *(apraxia)*.

Some children with a cleft palate have very unusual articulation patterns that are not seen in children who do not have cleft palate. These unusual articulations are called *compensatory misarticulations* or maladaptive articulations. They can be challenging to treat and require special speech therapy techniques. Surgery and orthodontics will not correct an articulation disorder.

Resonance disorders are seen in 20% to 30% of children born with a cleft palate. This occurs when the repaired palate is too short or does not move properly when the child speaks. It can also occur because of a hole (fistula) in the palate. Resonance disorders are physical problems, not learning problems. In these cases, air leaks through the child's nose during speech production. The air leakage can cause the child's speech to sound excessively nasal, or it might be audible when the child produces certain consonant sounds. Some children try to close off an air leak by scrunching their noses or face; this is called nasal or facial grimacing.

If no fistula is present in the palate, the problem that causes the resonance disorder is called velopharyngeal dysfunction, which is also called velopharyngeal insufficiency. Because it is a physical problem, it cannot be corrected with speech therapy. It is corrected with surgery or, less commonly, with a dental appliance called a prosthesis.

Resonance and articulation disorders can occur at the same time in the same child or they can occur separately. Some types of articulation errors can trick the listener's ear into thinking that a resonance disorder is present. A speech-language pathologist on a cleft team is the best person to be able to sort out these types of errors. Understanding the differences between these types of articulations is important in ensuring that the child gets the right type of treatment.

A small number of children born with a cleft palate have a language disorder. A language disorder or impairment might be related to difficulty hearing in the early months of life. A child with a language impairment may have difficulty learning to understand or speak words and using words correctly in phrases and sentences. A speech-language pathologist can test for a language disorder by using standardized tests. Such tests have been given to large groups of children of different ages. This helps to understand whether a child is having greater difficulty than other children of the same age. Language disorders are occasionally diagnosed in children born with a cleft lip only or in children with various syndromes or neurologic impairment.

Occasionally, a child is diagnosed with a voice disorder. This can be caused by a physical problem or misuse of the *larynx* (voice box). Children with a voice disorder might have a hoarse voice or a breathy voice. This is diagnosed based on a careful evaluation by a speech-language pathologist and an examination of the voice box in which a special telescope is used to look through the child's mouth or nose. Depending on the findings, a voice disorder might be treated with speech therapy, medically, or both. It may or may not be related to the cleft palate.

Stuttering, or fluency disorder, is rare in children with a cleft palate. Stuttering is probably not related to the cleft. It is treated by a speech-language pathologist who specializes in fluency disorder.

A child with a cleft might have only one type of disorder or a combination of disorders. Every child with a cleft palate is unique, and no two children born with this difference have the same speech disorders. Articulation disorders in these children can occur in particular patterns. The cleft team speech-language pathologist can help to identify these patterns and effective treatment methods.

THE TIMING OF SPEECH THERAPY

Speech therapy should begin as soon as it is clear that the child has a speech or language disorder of some kind. Speech-language pathologists are familiar with normal speech development and can determine whether the child's speech development is different enough from that of other children to require therapy. Parents should ask the speech-language pathologist what type of speech disorder their child has developed.

Some children shows signs of an articulation disorder at approximately age 18 to 22 months, but they may not be developmentally ready for the structured therapy that is needed. The speech-language pathologist might suggest waiting a short time before starting therapy. Many children are ready for a structured therapy approach by their second birthday. Some cleft palate speech specialists prefer to wait until the child is 2½ to 3 years of age. This depends on the therapist's preferred techniques or approaches.

Because only speech therapy will correct an articulation disorder, there is no benefit to waiting until after orthodontics or surgery to begin therapy. Alternatively, if the child's articulation was normal before surgery or orthodontics, it will remain normal. It will not be necessary to resume speech therapy to relearn speech. The child will adjust to any changes in the mouth. If the child was in a speech therapy program at the time of surgery or orthodontics, this therapy should continue afterward.

THE NEED FOR A SPECIALIZED SPEECH-LANGUAGE PATHOLOGIST

In the United States, speech-language pathologists are not required to have course work or practical training in treating children with cleft palate speech. This is also true in some other countries. Very few speech-language pathologists have experience with cleft palate speech therapy. Parents should ask the speech therapist if he or she has training in cleft palate speech (see the section Important Information to Obtain From the Speech-Language Pathologist).

ENSURING APPROPRIATE SPEECH THERAPY FOR CHILDREN WHO LIVE FAR FROM A CLEFT TEAM

Communication between the cleft team speech-language pathologist and the speech-language pathologist close to home is essential. Parents should ask their child's therapist to send reports and contact the team speech-language pathologist. Some cleft palate medical teams offer collaborative care in which the local speech-language pathologist attends a special speech visit at the cleft center with the parents and their child. The local and team speech-language pathologists listen together, agree on what they are hearing, discuss or try different therapy techniques to determine what works best for the child, and develop a treatment plan. Usually, the parents sign a release for ongoing phone or email communication between the two speech-language pathologists. The speech-language pathologist at the medical center will bill the insurance company for a speech evaluation.

Collaborative care is focused on the child's needs. There are numerous types of cleft palate speech disorders. Every child is unique, and the therapy techniques that one child needs may be different from the needs of another child with cleft palate. When the team and local speech-language pathologists collaborate, they can provide services that fit every child's needs.

When collaborative care is not available, parents can refer to books and continuing education products that are designed specifically for cleft palate speech therapy. These can be purchased through professional associations and therapy materials suppliers and publishers. National and regional associations of speech-language pathologists in most countries hold annual meetings and conventions. Often, the speech-language pathologist can attend seminars and lectures on cleft palate speech therapy offered at these meetings.

IMPORTANT INFORMATION TO OBTAIN FROM THE SPEECH-LANGUAGE PATHOLOGIST

Parents should gather as much information as possible from the medical professionals who are helping their child. They should ask the speech-language pathologist the following questions:

- Do you have training in cleft palate speech therapy? Have you provided speech therapy to other children with cleft palate? Although most speech-language pathologists have limited training or experience in this area, they can nevertheless be good therapists.
- Are you willing to communicate and collaborate with the cleft team's speech-language pathologist? Parents should ask for a release form to sign giving permission for communication and give the speech-language pathologist the contact information for the team. Parents need to ask the speech-language pathologist to send the evaluation report and periodic progress reports to the team.
- What type of disorder or disorders have you identified? What treatment techniques do you plan to use?
- Will my child be seen individually or in a group for therapy? If the therapy is conducted in a group, how many other children will be in the group? Will all of the children will be working on similar things? Are they all getting the same type of therapy? How will you ensure that my child's needs will be met during the entire group therapy time?
- What can I do to help my child at home? Will you provide a home program with activities that I can do between therapy sessions? A home program is a valuable tool to help the child's speech therapy progress more quickly.

COMMUNICATING WITH THE CHILD'S SPEECH-LANGUAGE PATHOLOGIST AT SCHOOL

The school speech-language pathologist will write an individualized educational plan (IEP) for the child. It will include the goals of therapy and detail how much time per week or month the child will receive in therapy. Parents should attend the annual IEP meeting, where they will have the opportunity to ask questions, contribute to the goal-setting process, and communicate with therapists and teachers at their child's school. Periodic reports should be sent home, ideally each quarter or semester.

Parents need to discuss ways of communicating more frequently with the speech-language pathologist. Some therapists ask parents to call if they have questions, and some send a notebook back and forth that parents can use to communicate.

The child's therapy can take place directly with the speech-language pathologist, or it can be conducted primarily with a speech aide or speech implementer. If the therapy will be conducted by a speech aide or implementer, parents should ask how often the speech-language pathologist will see their child. How closely is the aide or implementer supervised?

THE ROLE OF MUSCLE STRENGTHENING IN TREATING CLEFT PALATE SPEECH DISORDERS

A therapy program that uses straws, horns, and whistles for muscle strengthening will not help the child's speech. Children with a cleft palate speech disorder do not have muscle weakness; they have learned incorrect patterns for making consonant sounds. Speech therapy should focus on teaching the child to make sounds correctly and practicing them until they become a habit. Therapy continues until the child can make the sounds easily and automatically and does not have to think about it during speech production.

Some therapists might use a blowing activity with a tube or air paddle to help teach a particular consonant, but this should not continue for weeks or months. Once the child can produce the target consonant, therapy should focus on habituating that consonant; blowing on an object is no longer needed.

Some therapists use nonspeech oral motor exercises. These include blowing, sucking, gagging, wagging the tongue back and forth outside the mouth, pushing the tongue into the cheeks, puckering the lips, lip and tongue popping, stretching to touch the nose or chin with the tongue tip, and other activities to wake up the mouth or to increase oral awareness. There is no evidence that these exercises offer any benefit. It is better to teach the child the names for the parts of the mouth or other words that will be used to teach speech sounds.

CONCLUSION

Speech therapy is a very important piece of the child's cleft treatment program. It should be provided by a speech-language pathologist trained in cleft-related speech disorders who is in communication with the cleft team. Parents who have questions about their child's therapy program should talk with the child's therapist directly. The cleft team's speech-language pathologist is another valuable resource. A release should be signed allowing the team and community speech-language pathologists to talk directly with one another for the best possible coordination. With a strong speech therapy program and an emphasis on communication between the family and the child's cleft team and local speech therapists, excellent speech outcomes can be expected.

14

Hearing Disorders

Noel Jabbour

KEY POINTS

○ Children with cleft palate are at high risk for *middle-ear disease* and hearing loss from accumulation of middle-ear fluid.

○ Hearing loss that results from fluid in the middle-ear can be managed with placement of a ventilation tube *(tympanostomy tube)* in the eardrum.

○ Other forms of hearing loss can be present in children with cleft palates who have other craniofacial syndromes.

○ Frequent evaluation of the ears and hearing is recommended for all patients with cleft palate.

W‌e are exposed to a symphony of sounds before we are born, from the sound of our mother's heartbeat to the voices of our family discussing plans for our arrival. After birth, the ability to hear is a vital part of understanding the world around us.

All noise involves waves of sound that create vibrations in the air. The ear consists of three parts: the outer ear, the middle ear, and the inner ear (Fig. 14-1). For normal hearing to occur, the sound waves must travel through the outer ear. The vibrations then have to be transmitted through the middle ear and the inner ear, where the signal that a noise has been sensed begins its journey to the brain.

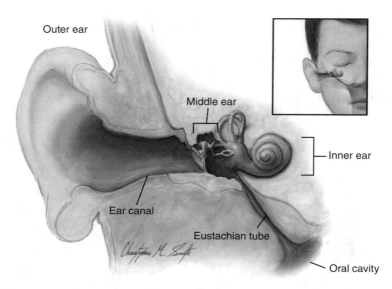

Fig. 14-1   The ear is composed of three parts: the outer ear, the middle ear, and the inner ear. The Eustachian tube connects the middle ear to the upper part of the throat, near the back of the nose.

The outer ear consists of the portion of the ear that can be seen from the outside *(pinna),* including the ear canal to the level of the *eardrum,* which is known as the *tympanic membrane.* The eardrum is the boundary between the outer ear and the middle ear. When the sound waves vibrate the eardrum, small bones in the middle ear called *ossicles* amplify the vibrations. There are three ossicles, named after their shapes: the malleus (the hammer), the incus (the anvil), and the stapes (the stirrup). Amazingly, because of the size and shape of the eardrum and the ossicles, these structures act as an amplification system to increase the vibration of sound that is presented to the inner ear.

The stapes bone is the final step of this vibration pathway in the middle ear; it is positioned at the boundary between the middle ear and the inner ear. The stapes perfectly fits and slides back and forth, like a piston, in a small opening called the *oval window.* The vibration of the stapes allows mechanical vibration of the ossicles to be transmitted to the fluids contained in the inner ear.

The inner ear consists of a spiral-shaped sound-sensing organ *(cochlea)* and organs that control balance. The cochlea contains thousands of sensors (hair cells) arranged according to frequency of vibrations that they sense. The hair cells are specially tuned to send a signal to the brain when they sense vibration. The precise location of these hair cells within the spiral shape of the cochlea allows us to discern sounds of different frequencies. Finally, from the hair cells, a signal is sent from the inner ear to the brain, where the sounds are processed.

EUSTACHIAN TUBE PROBLEMS AND CONDUCTIVE HEARING LOSS

The middle ear is normally filled with air because of a connection between the middle ear and the upper part of the throat, near the back of the nose, called the *Eustachian tube.* Normally, the Eustachian tube opens and closes in response to movement of the muscles of the palate. A particular muscle, the *levator veli palatini,* is involved in palate movement and is also responsible for opening the Eustachian tube. One end of this muscle is attached to the cartilage of the Eustachian tube, and the other end is attached in the midline of the palate, to its corresponding muscle on the opposite side. These muscles pull against each other to open the Eustachian tube as well as elevating the soft palate for speech.

In patients with a cleft palate, the muscles on each side of the palate cannot pull against each other properly, and their function in opening the Eustachian tube is compromised. When this occurs, the middle ear can develop a negative pressure, like a low-pressure vacuum. This negative pressure increases the likelihood of middle-ear infections and fluid or mucus accumulation in the middle-ear space; this is known as *middle-ear effusion.*

The normal hearing pathway relies on the amplification system provided by the eardrum and the ossicles. For this amplification system to work, the eardrum and the ossicles need to move freely in the air space of the middle ear without any restriction. Just as it is easier to walk on the sand at the beach than to walk through the water, it is easier for the ossicles to move when surrounded by air than when submerged in fluid. Any dampening of this system, for example, by middle-ear effusion, can lead to a problem in conducting sound waves to the inner ear; this type of hearing loss is called a *conductive hearing loss.*

When a cleft palate is unrepaired, the levator veli palatine muscles cannot function properly. In these patients, the rate of Eustachian tube dysfunction has been estimated to be 80% to 90%. This rate drops to 40% to 60% after the palate has been repaired. Patients with *Eustachian tube dysfunction* and middle-ear effusion commonly have a degree of hearing loss of approximately 20 decibels (dB)—about the same amount of loss that occurs by plugging the ear canals with the fingers.

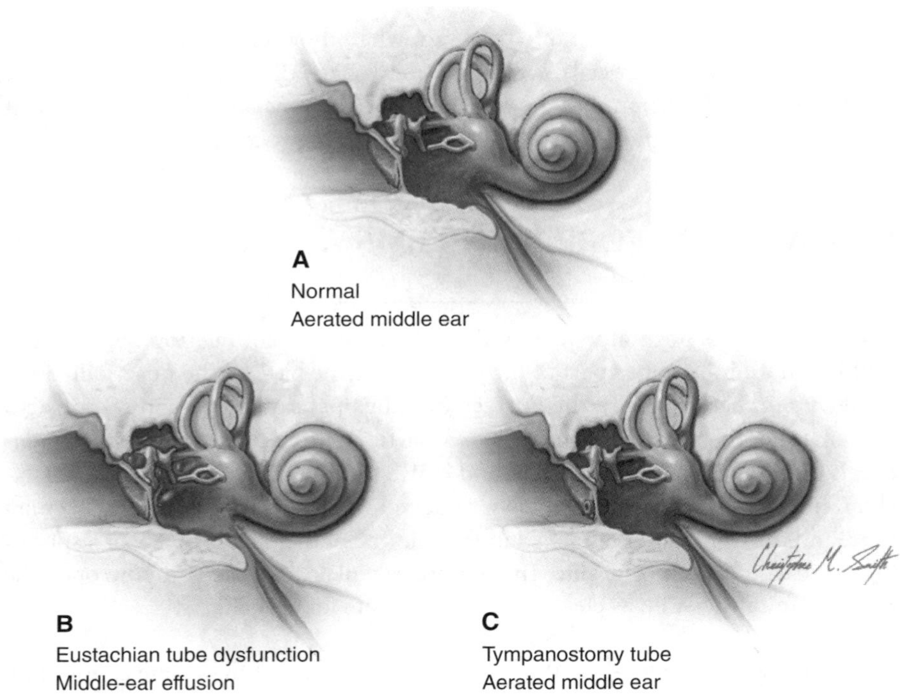

A
Normal
Aerated middle ear

B
Eustachian tube dysfunction
Middle-ear effusion

C
Tympanostomy tube
Aerated middle ear

Fig. 14-2   Close-up view of the middle ear in three different states. **A,** Normal aerated middle ear. **B,** Eustachian tube dysfunction with middle-ear effusion (fluid accumulation). **C,** Tympanostomy tube in place in aerated middle ear.

With surgical closure of the palate, management of the ear disease, and improvement in the anatomy with growth, most children with a cleft palate have normal hearing and less difficulty with Eustachian tube dysfunction by 6 years of age. For some, however, Eustachian tube dysfunction can be a lifelong process.

Treatment for Eustachian Tube Dysfunction

A common treatment for Eustachian tube dysfunction is surgical placement of pressure equalization tubes (tympanostomy tubes) in the eardrums. While the patient is under anesthesia, generally at the time of cleft lip or cleft palate repair, each eardrum is viewed with a microscope. A small incision is made in the eardrum, and the fluid in the middle ear is removed with suctioning. This allows the middle ear to be filled with air again. To continue to ensure that the middle ear remains aerated, a small tympanostomy tube is placed to span the incision that was made in the eardrum. This tube allows long-term ventilation between the middle ear and the outer ear. It provides the air needed in the middle ear for proper movement of the eardrum and ossicles. It also allows topical antibiotic eardrops to be placed in the middle ear for treatment of future middle-ear infections, as an alternative to giving oral antibiotics.

OTHER CAUSES OF HEARING LOSS

Some patients have hearing loss from causes other than Eustachian tube dysfunction, especially patients whose cleft palate is part of a syndrome. For example, a patient might have an additional conductive loss, or a hearing loss that results from of a problem transmitting the signal from the inner ear to the brain. This type of hearing loss is called a *sensorineural hearing loss.* Some patients have a conductive hearing loss and a sensorineural hearing loss.

Certain syndromes that include cleft palate can involve problems in the development of the outer ear, middle ear, or inner ear. Issues of the outer ear might involve a small ear, a malformed ear, or an absent ear, all of which are called *microtia.* These patients can have a narrow or absent ear canal and underdevelopment of the middle-ear structures. This anatomic difference is known as *aural atresia* and can cause a significant conductive hearing loss.

All newborns need to have their hearing screened shortly after birth. If this hearing screening is not passed, it is important to follow up with an *audiologist* for secondary testing. If secondary testing indicates a possible hearing loss, a referral should be made to an *otolaryngologist* for further diagnosis and treatment. Some patients need to use hearing aids. Patients born with a cleft palate have a higher risk of Eustachian tube dysfunction and other delayed causes of hearing loss and should have regular hearing assessments, even if they pass the newborn hearing screening.

COMMON HEARING TESTS

Generally, the first-line hearing screening performed at birth is called *otoacoustic emissions,* or OAE. This test relies on the principle that the small hair cells in the cochlea of the inner ear produce a very quiet noise that can be captured by a very sensitive microphone placed in the ear canal. In a patient with a healthy middle ear and functioning inner ear, this noise will be transmitted, and the patient will pass the screening.

For children who do not pass repeated OAE testing, a second-line test can be performed, called an *auditory brainstem response,* or ABR. In this test, a sound is presented to the patient's ear, and the brain activity is measured along different aspects of the neural signal. The ABR can provide reliable estimates of hearing sensitivity across the frequency range. This test is best performed when the child is asleep. It is often performed in young infants while they are napping, but older children might require a medicine for sedation.

Beginning around 6 months of age, children may be able to reliably participate in behavioral testing of hearing. For these younger infants, visual reinforcement audiometry, or VRA, can be performed. This test measures the sound levels needed to produce a behavioral response, such as a head turn toward a visually interesting display (video or lighted toy), that occurs immediately after a sound is presented from the same direction. This is a form of conditioning in which a child is rewarded with a visual display after the behavioral response to the noise. If a child can tolerate headphones, ear-specific information can be obtained. If not, speakers can be used to obtain non-ear-specific information.

Around 2 years of age, children may begin to tolerate testing that involves performing certain tasks with toys or puzzles in response to sounds, such as placing a ball in a basket when a tone is heard. This is called play audiometry.

Tympanometry is a test that evaluates eardrum mobility in response to changes in air pressure presented through the ear canal. This test is used to infer middle-ear function and to determine whether the eardrum mobility is (A) normal, (B) reduced because of fluid in the middle ear or a hole in the eardrum, or (C) abnormal from negative pressure in the middle ear. When combined with a careful examination of the ear, tympanometry can help clinicians determine middle-ear function with good reliability.

CONCLUSION

Nearly all infants with cleft palates have Eustachian tube dysfunction, which may lead to middle-ear effusions and conductive hearing loss. For patients with prolonged middle-ear effusions or conductive hearing loss, tympanostomy tubes may need to be placed. This is generally done at the time of lip repair or palate repair. Because of the higher risk of middle-ear disease and hearing loss in children with a cleft palate, frequent follow-up visits for ear evaluation and hearing assessment are recommended.

15

Diagnostic Audiology

Diane L. Sabo

KEY POINTS

o Hearing loss should be diagnosed during newborn screenings.

o The severity of hearing loss may change over time.

o Hearing loss can be caused by different problems.

o Cleft palate anatomy can cause hearing loss.

o Hearing is very important in learning and development.

Hearing loss can be a lifelong disability. It can alter the development of speech, language, and cognition in children, especially when it occurs early in life. In addition, other areas may be affected, including academic achievement and social and emotional development. Hearing loss is often misunderstood; the lack of response to sounds and delays in development is frequently attributed to other causes. Not only the person with the hearing loss is affected, but also others in the person's environment.

Early detection and intervention can decrease or possibly eliminate poor outcomes. Treatment might include hearing aids and educational support and services. Studies have shown that early intervention can help to achieve communication skills comparable to those of children of the same age who have no hearing loss.

Approximately two or three in every 1000 children are born with hearing loss in the United States. Approximately 8000 to 12,000 babies are born each year with permanent hearing loss, most of whom have parents who can hear. Congenital hearing loss is more common than other conditions for which newborns are routinely screened.

The number of children with hearing loss increases and is nearly doubled in children of school age—5 in every 1000 children 3 to 17 years of age. This number increases as the population ages. Today, approximately 36 million adult Americans (17%) report some degree of hearing loss. In addition, three of four children have an ear infection (otitis media) by the time they are 3 years of age. (This can cause hearing loss and is discussed later in the chapter.)

HEARING SCREENING

The age at which infants and children are diagnosed with a hearing loss has changed significantly in the past 10 years because of universal newborn hearing screening (UNHS). Hearing loss is identified at earlier ages than it was previously. Before routine newborn hearing screening for all infants was performed, the average age of identification of hearing loss was 2 years. With newborn hearing screening, it is identified before children are 6 months of age.

Screening for hearing loss is recommended for all newborns by 1 month of age. If a baby does not pass the newborn screening, the next step is a complete hearing assessment, which is known as diagnostic audiology testing. The initial diagnostic tests must be completed as soon as possible to diagnose potential hearing loss before the child is 3 months of age. A baby identified with a hearing loss should be fit with hearing aids (if appropriate) and enrolled in an early intervention program well before 6 months of age. These guidelines, commonly referred to as the 1-3-6 model, have been widely adopted by many national organizations.

Periodic hearing (audiologic) examinations of infants are recommended to detect later-onset hearing loss. Some conditions can cause hearing loss to get worse over time (progressive), whereas others cause hearing loss when the child is older (delayed-onset hearing loss). Children with these conditions should be referred for an audiologic assessment at least once by 24 to 30 months of age. Children at risk for delayed-onset hearing loss, such as those with cytomegalovirus infection, should have more frequent audiologic assessments. The Joint Committee on Infant Hearing provides a list of conditions that can be associated with progressive or delayed onset of hearing loss in childhood.

DEVELOPMENT OF AUDITORY BEHAVIOR

Infants are born with the ability to hear. As they age, changes occur in their awareness of sound, their connections to the brain in the nervous system, and the way their central nervous system uses auditory information. The changes in the central nervous system continue to develop well into childhood and adolescence. During pregnancy, the auditory system becomes functional at the end of the second trimester or during the third trimester, at approximately week 25 of gestation.

Early in life, infants respond to sound in a reflexive manner until they develop the motor control for more organized responses. As infants get older, they respond to a decreased level of the sound. More specifically, their hearing does not improve with age, but they begin to pay attention to softer sounds. We can measure their attention to these sounds more easily and consistently as they get older.

Infants begin to identify the location or direction of where sounds originate. This is known as localization. It occurs first in horizontal (left to right) and then vertical planes (up and down). From 3 to 6 months of age, infants search for the sound, respond to the sound of their name, and respond differently depending on the parent's tone of voice. By 5 to 6 months of age, formal and reliable behavioral audiologic testing can begin (see Behavioral Audiometry later in the chapter). From 6 to 10 months of age, infants can seek out the source of sound and respond to common sounds in their environment. They respond to loud and soft sounds and pay attention when their parent talks to them. From 10 to 15 months of age, babbling increases and begins to more closely resemble speech. From 15 to 18 months of age, young children are able to identify the origin of most sounds, understand simple phrases, identify familiar objects such as body parts, and follow simple directions. By 18 months of age, children should have a vocabulary of 20 or more words and short phrases.

HOW WE HEAR

The Ear

The ear has three main parts: the outer ear, the middle ear, and the inner ear (Fig. 15-1). Each part has a specific function in sound detection. Hearing loss can occur when any part of the hearing system does not work in the usual way.

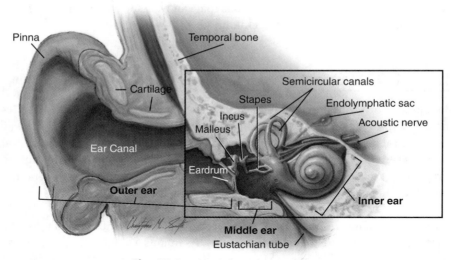

Fig. 15-1   The three parts of the ear.

The three parts of the ear are made up of the following structures:
1. *Outer ear*
   - The pinna is the part we see on the sides of the head
   - The ear canal leads to the eardrum.
   - The eardrum (tympanic membrane) separates the outer and middle ear.
2. *Middle ear*
   - The eardrum separates the outer and middle ear.
   - The space behind the eardrum contains air and the ossicles.
   - Three small bones called ossicles are located in the space behind the eardrum. These are the malleus, incus, and stapes, commonly referred to as the hammer, anvil, and stirrup.
3. *Inner ear*
   - The cochlea senses sound vibrations and transmits the signal to the brain.
   - The semicircular canals help to control balance.

Acoustic Nerve

Sound waves follow a specific pathway through the ear to reach the acoustic nerve, which sends sound information from the inner ear to the brain. Sound waves travel through the outer ear and cause the vibration of the eardrum and the ossicles in the middle ear. This, in turn, leads to movement of fluid in the inner ear, which moves tiny hairs in the cochlea of the inner ear. This fluid and hair cell movement triggers the acoustic nerve to send the signal to the brain. The brain receives the message and identifies it as sound.

TYPES OF HEARING LOSS

Hearing losses can be located in the external ear, the middle ear, the inner ear, or in a combination of these locations. It can also occur in the nerve pathway from the inner ear to the brain. The specific location determines the type of hearing loss, which are described in Table 15-1.

Hearing loss is classified in many ways. The following descriptors are common:
- Unilateral or bilateral: Hearing loss is in one ear (unilateral) or both ears (bilateral).
- Prelingual or postlingual: Hearing loss happens before the child learns to talk (prelingual) or after the child learns to talk (postlingual).
- Symmetrical or asymmetrical: Hearing loss is the same in both ears (symmetrical) or is different in each ear (asymmetrical).
- Progressive or sudden onset: Hearing loss worsens over time (progressive) or happens quickly (sudden onset).
- Fluctuating or stable: Hearing loss gets better and worse over time (fluctuating) or stays the same over time (stable).
- Congenital or acquired (delayed) onset: Hearing loss is present at birth (congenital) or develops later in life (acquired or delayed onset).

Table 15-1   Types of Hearing Loss

Type of Hearing Loss	Cause	Treatment
Conductive hearing loss	Caused by something that stops some or all sounds from passing through the outer and/or middle ear. Sound is not directed properly to the inner ear. Common causes are excessive wax in the outer ear, a middle-ear infection, and fluid in the middle ear.	Most types of conductive hearing loss can be treated medically or surgically and are more often temporary.
Sensorineural hearing loss	Caused by damage to the inner ear (sensory) or acoustic nerve (neural). Common causes of this type of loss in young children are differences in the structures of the inner ear, specific types of illness that occur before birth, lack of oxygen during birth, genetic or inherited factors, and specific drugs.	This hearing loss cannot be cured medically or surgically and is permanent.
Auditory neuropathy	Caused by a nerve that cannot send the signal to the brain in the same manner that a healthy nerve does. Children with this hearing loss show a variety of responses to sounds and variability in speech and language development.	This type of hearing loss is more common in infants born prematurely.
Mixed hearing loss	Caused by a combination of conductive and sensorineural hearing loss. For example, children with sensorineural hearing loss can develop ear infections (fluid in the middle ear) that can make the hearing worse during the time that fluid is present.	Some components of mixed hearing loss may be treatable.

DEGREES OF HEARING LOSS

Hearing is measured in decibels (dB). A value of 0 dB is the reference value at which young adults with normal hearing detect a tone of a given intensity (loudness) and frequency (pitch) half of the time. There is no single standard for determining the degree (severity) of hearing loss. For children, the classification of the degree of hearing loss is often strict, because hearing loss in infants and young children can significantly affect the development of speech and language. This can result in negative educational consequences if left undetected and untreated. At average conversational levels, the sound of several consonants (s, p, k, th, f, and sh) is at or below normal hearing levels in adults. A hearing ability better than 20 to 25 dB is needed for more consistent detection of these sounds. This is the reason the critical range of normal hearing is set at 0 to 15 dB for young children.

A common classification system for hearing loss in children is the following:
- Normal range (-10 to 15 dB)
- Slight hearing loss (16 to 25 dB)
- Mild hearing loss (26 to 40 dB)
- Moderate hearing loss (41 to 55 dB)
- Moderately severe hearing loss (56 to 70 dB)
- Severe hearing loss (71 to 90 dB)
- Profound hearing loss (91+ dB)

Another way to define hearing loss is to use more functional descriptions such as hard of hearing and deaf. The term hard of hearing refers to people with hearing loss who can hear to some degree, whereas deafness typically involves complete inability to hear. Children who are hard of hearing learn language primarily through hearing. Someone who is functionally deaf learns primarily visually; methods of visual learning include lip reading, manual communication, and sign language.

CLEFT PALATE AND HEARING LOSS

Children with a cleft need to have audiologic testing as soon as possible. The American Cleft Palate-Craniofacial Association recommends that they have this test within the first 3 months of age to obtain a baseline of their hearing because of their increased risk of conductive and sensorineural hearing loss. Conductive hearing losses may come and go (for example, worsening during episodes of middle-ear problems), or they can be permanent structural malformations of the ear. Sensorineural hearing loss and cleft palate occur together in several syndromes involving the head and neck. For example, children with Treacher Collins syndrome and *Nager syndrome* can have structural ear problems and cleft palate. Other syndromes associated with a cleft palate can cause conductive hearing loss from middle-ear fluid or other structural anomalies.

Fluid collection in the middle ear can lead to middle-ear infections, which can eventually cause conductive hearing loss. Children with a cleft palate frequently have fluid collection in the middle ear and middle-ear infections because of Eustachian tube dysfunction, which may or may not resolve after cleft palate repair. The Eustachian tube connects the middle ear with the back of the throat and allows fresh air to enter the middle-ear space (see Chapter 14). The fresh air helps to maintain proper pressure in the middle ear and keeps the middle ear free of fluid. A cleft palate can prevent the muscles that open the Eustachian tube from working properly. Therefore the tube itself does not work properly.

Management

A middle-ear infection generally causes a mild-to-moderate conductive hearing loss, although not everyone with a middle-ear infection will have a hearing loss. Aggressive management is needed to minimize the amount of time that middle-ear fluid (and possibly conductive hearing loss) is present. Antibiotics are a common treatment. Another common treatment is a *myringotomy* with tympanostomy tube insertion. A myringotomy is a tiny incision made in the eardrum to relieve pressure and to drain fluid from the middle ear. A small tube (tympanostomy tube) is inserted into the eardrum to keep the middle ear ventilated. Tympanostomy tubes can become blocked and/or fall out, requiring reinsertion. Surgery to repair the cleft palate often helps with drainage of middle-ear fluid, but drainage may not occur immediately after cleft repair. Therefore a myringotomy with tympanostomy tube insertion is often performed during or after the cleft surgery.

On average, hearing loss caused by middle-ear fluid collections and infection usually resolves by the time children are 5 years old. This age is consistent with the age when Eustachian tube dysfunction usually resolves (5 to 6 years of age in 75% to 94% of children affected). However, some children (2% to 24%) have persistent hearing loss after 5 to 6 years of age. Persistent hearing loss in children with a repaired cleft palate has been attributed to postoperative scarring and poor movement of the palate, and can be addressed if necessary.

A high percentage of children with cleft palate have middle-ear fluid collections and infections. For this reason, some physicians routinely place tympanostomy tubes to try to ensure good hearing during critical periods of speech and language development. Medical professionals are not all in agreement regarding routine placement of tympanostomy tubes.

SPECIFIC AUDIOLOGIC TESTS

Newborn Hearing Screening

Newborn hearing screening is usually conducted while the newborn is in the hospital after birth. Several organizations have recommended using two different tests: otoacoustic emissions (OAEs) and auditory brainstem response (ABR). These tests do not require participation from the infant.

Otoacoustic Emissions

When the cochlea works normally, it receives sound and produces very soft measurable sounds called OAEs. For this test, a small earpiece is placed into the infant's ear. Sounds are presented to the child, and the very soft measurable sounds produced by the child's cochlea are recorded with a microphone that is in the earpiece. The soft sounds travel through the middle ear to get to the microphone. Therefore a requirement of the test is that the middle ear be clear of fluid.

Auditory Brainstem Response

ABR testing measures how the inner ear and/or auditory nerve respond to sounds. Electrodes or sensors are placed on the infant's head and/or neck, and sounds are presented to the ear. The electrodes detect the nerve activity. Generally, infants younger than 6 months of age do not need sedation for this test. For older children and those who do not sleep well and need sedation, ABR testing is conducted in a special clinic room or hospital operating room. In either case, a physician must be on site, and a medical professional must monitor the infant's vital signs (heart rate, breathing rate, temperature, and blood pressure) during the test.

Some recommend that an OAE test be performed first, followed by an ABR test if the OAE results are not normal. However, hospital personnel can use whatever method or methods they choose. Many people think that children with a cleft palate will fail their newborn screenings, because middle-ear fluid collections, conductive hearing loss, and sensorineural hearing loss are more common in these children. There is little evidence showing this to be true.

Regardless of newborn hearing screening outcomes, all children with a cleft palate should be seen regularly, because they have a high risk of middle-ear fluid collections and infection. Furthermore, children who are at risk for fluctuating or changing losses need to be seen regularly to monitor the changes over time.

The same tests used for screening are used in the audiology follow-up, especially for young infants. Screening tests are often automated so that they can be performed by a trained technician. This is not the case for diagnostic testing. The diagnostic evaluation is performed by a pediatric audiologist, or an expert in hearing with the necessary skills to test infants and young children. The audiologist performs a series of tests to determine whether the child has a hearing loss. If a loss is confirmed, the type (the part of the auditory system affected), the degree (how much hearing loss exists), and the configuration (the frequencies or pitches that are affected) of the loss are also determined.

Several tests are needed to thoroughly evaluate the type and amount of hearing loss in an infant or young child. For very young patients, we rely on tests that do not require the baby to show responses to sounds (for example, the ABR screen), because they are not capable of providing valid behavioral indications of hearing. As children get older and have more consistent responses to sounds, the ABR screen is not done as often, and tests that assess behavioral responses are performed. The age at which these tests can be given depends on each child's development. They are reliable in some children who are younger than 1 year of age.

The following tests are performed to evaluate infants for hearing loss. Some are also performed as screening tests.

Auditory Steady State Responses

Auditory steady state response (ASSR) testing is another measurement of a baby's hearing that does not rely on the baby responding to sound. The benefit of ASSR testing is that the sounds can be made louder than the sounds used with the ABR screen; therefore this test may provide more information for infants who have severe to profound hearing loss. This information can help the audiologist to better understand the hearing loss to determine whether a hearing aid or a *cochlear implant* is needed. Currently, ASSR is not available in all audiologic clinics and is used to supplement ABR test results. Infants older than 6 months of age may need to be sedated for ASSR testing.

Tympanometry

Tympanometry assesses the condition of the middle ear. An earpiece similar to the one used for OAE testing is placed in the ear, and air pressure changes are made in the ear canal. For infants less than 6 months of age, specialized equipment generating a high-frequency tone is needed, because very young infants have small, soft ear canals that can affect the test and give inaccurate results. Using the specialized equipment increases the reliability and accuracy of tympanometry for children 0 to 6 months of age.

Behavioral Audiometry

Hearing tests use behavioral measures for children with a developmental age of approximately 6 months. During testing, the audiologist finds the lowest intensity (loudness) level at which a child can detect sound at different frequencies (pitches). The hearing information for the lowest intensity levels for each frequency is plotted on a graph called an audiogram. Similar to adult hearing testing, behavioral testing of infants is conducted in a sound-treated room or a soundproof booth. Behavioral response levels can be obtained using visual reinforcement audiometry (VRA), play audiometry, and conventional audiometry for older children. VRA and play audiometry are adaptations of traditional hearing test methods (conventional audiometry). The results are reliable and valid when the tests are conducted by experienced audiologists.

Visual Reinforcement Audiometry

VRA is recommended for children 6 to 30 months of age. The infant or young child is seated on a caregiver's lap or in a high chair in a soundproof booth. The child is trained to turn the head, either toward a moving toy or video screen that lights up, each time a sound is heard. Individual ears are tested with earphones and other instruments, and the results are plotted on an audiogram. If the child is reluctant to wear earphones, the sounds can be presented through speakers; this is called sound field testing. Although better cooperation is sometimes possible when earphones are not worn, information about the hearing levels in each ear separately cannot be determined when sound field testing is used.

Conditioned Play Audiometry

For children approximately 2½ years of age, testing can usually be done using a play task called conditioned play audiometry (CPA). The child is taught to respond to tones by playing a simple game using toys such as stacking rings, peg boards, simple puzzles, or a combination of play activities to maintain interest. Each ear is tested separately with earphones and other instruments, and the results are plotted on an audiogram.

Conventional Audiometry

For children with a developmental age of approximately 5 years, conventional behavioral audiometry can be conducted using a hand-raise response. Testing methods may need to be changed to maintain the child's interest and participation.

Similar to testing of adults, speech is used as part of the evaluation for children with sufficient language skills, typically at the developmental age of 3 to 4 years. Adaptations are made to ensure that the child is able to participate in the task and that his or her attention can be maintained. The earliest speech testing often begins with pointing to an object and, for young children, advances to pointing to pictures. This progresses to saying words or sentences for children who have developed sufficient language.

REVIEWING TEST RESULTS

The pediatric audiologic evaluation often requires repeated visits scheduled close together to determine the exact details, the degree, and sometimes the nature of the hearing loss. It is a time-intensive and ongoing process, particularly for very young infants with a hearing loss.

Complete information about hearing at all frequencies (pitches) is the goal of testing and is needed to fit a hearing aid for patients with a permanent hearing loss. However, reliable estimates at critical frequencies can be used to start the process. Adjustments can be made as more information is obtained. Delays are not acceptable, even when only partial information is available.

HEARING AID FITTING

For children who have permanent sensorineural or conductive hearing loss, sounds need to be louder (amplified). This is usually done with personal hearing aids. The goal of hearing aids is to make the speech of others loud enough to be understood. Children learn spoken communication skills from hearing the sounds around them. The ability to hear consonant sounds is critical to understanding the spoken message. Advances in hearing aid technology have helped to produce better outcomes for children with hearing loss. In general, hearing aids have become smaller and fit better on small ears so that they stay on. More options and better strategies for enhancing spoken background sounds are available.

Similar to the evaluation, hearing aid fitting is a process. It is not accomplished in one visit. The child's ear does not reach adult size until nearly 9 years of age. Changes in growth and stiffness of the ear affect the output of the hearing aid: In general, smaller ears result in a higher intensity of sound. This output variability can be as high as 15 dB, resulting in uncomfortable or even damaging levels in a young child's ear. Because ears vary greatly in size, regardless of age, measurements of hearing aid output need to be made with the device in the ear. For young children, this can be a challenge. It requires that they remain still and not vocalize while measurements are obtained.

The behind-the-ear style of hearing aid is the most widely used for young children. It has greater flexibility in fitting children with all degrees of hearing loss and is durable. Moreover, cost is reduced, because only the earmold has to be replaced as the ear grows. The in-the-ear style of hearing aids must be entirely remade as the ear grows, and this is quite expensive. Therefore this style may be appropriate for older children. In-the-ear hearing aids cannot be used with some hearing assistive technology, such as frequency modulation (FM) systems used in classrooms. Because hearing aids amplify all sounds, noise is amplified along with speech. In the classroom, children with hearing loss often struggle to hear the teachers because of the high levels of background noise. The ability to hear and understand verbal information is important for learning. In FM systems, the teacher wears a microphone close to the mouth, and the speech signal is sent to the child's hearing aid. They are commonly used in classrooms and can be used at home. FM systems can use speakers that are portable or mounted in the classroom, potentially benefiting all children in the classroom. Other assistive technology is available. Some modern systems incorporate Bluetooth in cell phones and MP3 players.

The benefits of hearing with both ears include sound localization and a better ability to understand what is said in a noisy background. Thus hearing aids are fit to both ears whenever possible or until continued testing proves this to be harmful or of no real benefit.

As discussed already, a child with cleft palate is at risk for recurrent middle-ear disease. If the child also has a permanent hearing loss, hearing aid use can be especially challenging and the benefit diminished. Fluctuating conductive impairment (problems in the middle ear) in a child with a permanent hearing loss will result in the child not hearing the sound as loudly as needed to benefit from the hearing aid during times of ear disease. This can possibly cause the child to reject the aid. Drainage from the ear can block the sound from the aid, damage the hearing aid, or cause feedback (whistle) from the hearing aid by blocking the ear canal. Lack of air circulation in the ear when the hearing aid is in place can make external or middle-ear infections worse.

For children with permanent conductive losses and malformed outer ears that prevent the use of standard behind-the-ear aids, *bone conduction* hearing aids are appropriate. Often, when these children are approximately 5 to 7 years of age, they will receive devices affixed to the bone around the ear, such as bone-anchored hearing aids (for example, BAHA or Ponto). A newer device such as the Sophono implant uses a sealed titanium case that houses a magnet, which is implanted under the skin to hold the bone vibrator in place. For younger children, the use of a BAHA bone vibrator with a soft headband is an option, because it provides a good-quality signal. A bone conduction hearing aid may also be appropriate for children who have chronic drainage from their ears. Because an earmold is not placed in the ear, it allows better ventilation of the middle ear.

Behind-the-ear hearing aids are ideal for children with a sensorineural loss and should be fit as soon as the hearing loss is defined. However, diligent monitoring is needed because of the problems with middle-ear fluid and infection and possible additional intermittent conductive hearing loss. Ideally, a hearing aid with an active volume control should be fit. This device provides the option of additional amplification when an effusion is present in the middle ear.

CONCLUSION

For children with a cleft palate and hearing loss, a good working relationship with a team of medical professionals is essential to address the various problems and concerns that arise. A team approach helps to maximize a child's ability to learn. Pediatric audiologists in clinics and educational audiologists in schools are an integral part of the team.

Part IV

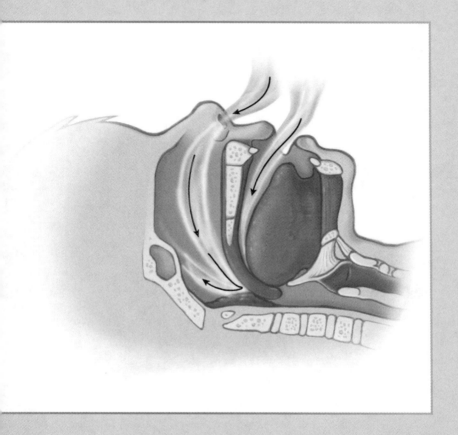

Airway and Breathing Issues

16

Pierre Robin Sequence

Matthew Greives

KEY POINTS

○ Pierre Robin sequence (PRS) consists of a group of related differences, including the following:
  - Micrognathia: A small jaw bone or mandible
  - Glossoptosis: A condition in which the tongue falls into the back of the throat, leading to breathing, swallowing, and feeding difficulties
  - Airway obstruction: Difficulty breathing caused by micrognathia and glossoptosis
  - Cleft palate: An opening in the palate that is often associated with PRS but is not a requirement for a diagnosis of PRS

○ Most cases of PRS occur randomly and are not caused by a genetic syndrome.

○ Infants with PRS are usually evaluated by a multidisciplinary team, which generally includes a plastic surgeon or jaw surgeon, an *ENT surgeon*, a speech and language therapist (specially trained in the assessment of swallowing), a neonatal critical care specialist (NICU [neonatal intensive care unit]), a genetics counselor (see Chapter 5), and a sleep specialist (see Chapter 17).

○ PRS can be mild to very severe. Different treatment options are available depending on the severity of the breathing difficulty.

P_{RS} was originally described by a French surgeon in 1923. He noted that infants born with a very small lower jaw (mandible) had extreme difficulty breathing. Often, these infants were unable to breathe on their own, because the amount of space in their mouth was small and their tongue fell to the back of their throat, causing obstruction. His original description of this sequence included micrognathia, *glossoptosis,* and breathing difficulty.

Unlike many conditions present at birth, PRS is a sequence not a syndrome. This means that the anatomic differences do not have a genetic cause in most patients. Many researchers believe that the small jaw is a result of the infant's face being compressed in the uterus during development, resulting in less growth of the mandible. However, genetic syndromes such as Treacher Collins and *Stickler syndrome* are associated with PRS. Therefore a team of genetic specialists must rule out these possible causes in every child diagnosed with PRS.

Infants with PRS were historically treated with a tracheostomy, or surgical airway created in the throat. Although this is still a treatment option, new advances in diagnosis and surgery have created better procedures for these children.

DIAGNOSIS AND WORKUP

The diagnosis of PRS is often made after birth. The pediatrician who performs the infant's first examination will notice the presence of the small jaw, which gives the facial profile a well recognizable appearance (Fig. 16-1). The pediatrician should also note any issues with breathing, swallowing, and feeding. These difficulties can include coughing, vomiting, gasping for air, unusual chest motion with breathing, and *cyanosis.* Oxygen monitors are used to assess the drop in the infant's oxygen level during feeding and sleeping. Often, these events are worse when the infant is in the *supine position,* because this causes the tongue to fall farther into the throat and block the airway. Sometimes, turning the infant over onto the stomach (prone) helps the tongue fall to the front of the mouth and makes breathing easier. In severe cases, a breathing tube is placed at birth to ensure that the infant is receiving adequate amounts of oxygen.

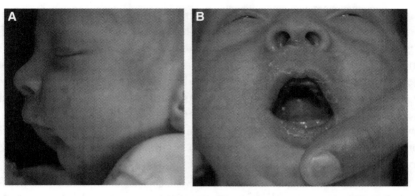

Fig. 16-1 An infant with Pierre Robin sequence. **A,** Note the small bottom jaw. **B,** The tip of the tongue can be seen within the cleft of the palate. Only the tip of the tongue is seen because the tongue has fallen backward (glossoptosis).

Infants diagnosed with PRS are usually transferred to the NICU for monitoring of the oxygen levels and a workup by the pediatric airway team. This team usually consists of the following:

- Genetics team: Performs the workup for genetic causes of PRS
- Neonatal intensive care specialist: Monitors infant's oxygen levels and coordinates care of other medical issues
- Sleep team: Analyzes the number of times the infant's oxygen level decreases during sleep
- Speech and swallow therapist: Evaluates the infant's risk for difficulty feeding, difficulty breathing, and *aspiration* of food into the trachea and lungs, rather than the stomach
- Surgeons: An ENT surgeon to evaluate the airway using nasal endoscopy, and a plastic or jaw surgeon to evaluate for surgical correction of the small jaw, tongue positioning, and cleft palate if present

During the workup for PRS, nasal endoscopy is one of the first examinations performed, and perhaps the most useful. The ENT surgeon and team will use an endoscope to look at the infant's airway. This instrument is a thin tube with a small camera attached to it. The endoscope is inserted into the infant's nostrils. The surgeon and team can assess the position of the tongue in relation to the back of the throat. In mild cases, the tongue falls back slightly into the airway and only partially obstructs the infant's ability to breath. In severe cases, the tongue falls all the way to the back of the throat, resulting in significant breathing difficulty. Sometimes, infants with severe obstruction need to have a breathing tube placed to ensure that their airway stays open.

A speech and swallow therapist will perform a bedside evaluation of the infant to measure the ability to swallow, feed, and breathe. Because of the pressure of the tongue on the back of the throat, many infants are unable to swallow normally. This can cause aspiration, which leads to coughing and gagging, increasing the risk for infection and damage in the lungs. If the findings of the evaluation are concerning, no feeding by mouth is allowed until the aspiration risks have been eliminated. The infant will be fed through a small feeding tube placed into the nose and passed down to the stomach. Many of these children have significant acid reflux from their stomach, which can cause aspiration. Most infants with PRS are given medicine shortly after birth to prevent acid reflux.

A genetics evaluation is a critical component of the workup for infants with PRS. Although most infants with PRS are otherwise normal and healthy, some have a genetic syndrome associated with the condition. The most common of these is Stickler syndrome, which is a genetic difference in the formation of collagen. Collagen is a component of many of the tissues in our bodies. A trained ophthalmologist can best diagnose Stickler syndrome with a thorough eye examination during the initial workup. Another syndrome, Treacher Collins, is associated with multiple other congenital differences in the face and skull. Blood can be drawn for genetic testing and analysis of other more rare syndromes. The team will counsel the parents about these diagnoses.

Most issues with breathing occur while the infant is asleep. The problems are worse when the infant sleeps on his or her back, because gravity can cause the tongue to fall back. A sleep study is performed to look at the number of times an infant's oxygen level decreases during sleep. In this study, multiple things are monitored, including the infant's oxygen and carbon dioxide levels, brain waves, and heart rate. Videos of the infant's positioning are recorded. A doctor trained in sleep medicine evaluates the results and counts the number of these events that occur over the course of the examination. This helps to gauge the severity of the breathing obstruction and guide the decision for surgical management.

A plastic or jaw surgeon, usually with a specialization in craniofacial surgery or pediatric plastic surgery, will examine the physical relationship of the jaw, tongue, and airway. In general, the farther back the lower jaw is positioned relative to the upper jaw, the worse the problem. A computed tomography scan is often performed. This is known as a CT scan. With this test, the surgeon can measure the size of the small mandible and plan for any surgery that may be necessary.

Once this information has been gathered, the team will sit down and discuss all of their individual findings and recommend treatment plans. Each patient has unique differences. With the team approach, all members contribute their considerations, and an appropriate treatment plan is developed that accounts for all aspects of the child's condition.

INTERVENTIONS

The degree of intervention in children with PRS depends on the severity of their symptoms. Many options are weighed for each infant, from nonsurgical measures to more invasive operations. There are two nonoperative options for infants with mild to moderate PRS: *prone positioning* and nasopharyngeal airway placement. For more severe cases of PRS, three surgical options are available: *tongue-lip adhesion,* mandibular distraction osteotomy (MDO), and tracheostomy.

Infants with a mild degree of airway obstruction can often be treated nonoperatively. As they get older, many of these children will "grow out of the condition," meaning, their lower jaw will grow sufficiently to allow them to breath and feed normally. Some of these infants will need to be maintained in a prone position while sleeping to ensure the best position of their tongue. During prone positioning, the oxygen levels should be continuously monitored. *Apnea* monitors are alarms that measure the infant's breathing and alert parents if the oxygen levels become too low. These monitors are used continuously at home until a repeat sleep study demonstrates that oxygen levels remain normal while the infant sleeps.

In children with a mild to moderate amount of airway obstruction, a nasopharyngeal (NP) airway can be placed in the nostril and advanced to the back of the throat to maintain an open passageway for breathing. This small rubber tube is left in the infant's nose and can push the tongue up and off the back of the throat to allow air to pass through normally. Similar to prone positioning, this is a temporary measure that can be continued while the infant's jaw grows. Most institutions will keep the child in the hospital for monitoring until oxygen levels are normal without the NP airway. Most infants are irritated by the NP airway initially, but tolerate it well after it has been placed. While the NP airway is in place, the infant is maintained in the prone position and wears an oxygen monitor at all times.

For infants with more severe airway obstruction, surgery to correct the unusual tongue position or small jaw size may be indicated. In infants with a significant degree of glossoptosis and those whose tongue falls back into their throat, a tongue-lip adhesion can be performed if the jaw is nearly normal. In this surgery, a small incision is made underneath the tongue and another incision is made inside the lower lip. A suture is then placed to create an adhesion or attachment between the tip of the tongue and the lip. This pulls the tongue forward and prevents it from dropping into the throat and blocking the passageway. The procedure is performed in the operating room while the patient is under general anesthesia. After surgery, the infant is monitored in the NICU. The breathing tube remains in place for a while so that the tongue-lip adhesion heals. After the infant has grown sufficiently and the airway risk has decreased, another surgery is performed to release the adhesion. The child's tongue and lip are usually normal after this surgery.

In many centers MDO is becoming the mainstay of treatment for children with PRS. Since its recent invention, it has grown in popularity because of its powerful ability to grow new bone in the small mandible and improve the airway. The child is under general anesthesia for this procedure. A small incision is made under the jaw on both sides of the infant's neck. Through this small incision, the mandible is cut to separate the front of the jaw from the back of the jaw. A distraction device is then placed over this cut in the bone and secured with small screws. Small metal pins, attached to the device, are then placed through the skin and remain outside the neck. All the incisions are closed and the infant is taken back to the NICU with the breathing tube in place. Starting soon after surgery, the pins are turned a few times every day. The pins are attached to a crank on the distractor device that slowly widens the device and separates the cut in the mandible. As the cut in the bone widens, new bone forms in the space and effectively increases the length of the mandible. Because the tongue is attached to the bottom jaw (a normal attachment), this movement pulls the tongue out of the throat and opens the airway. After a few days, when the swelling from surgery has resolved and the jaw has grown sufficiently, the breathing tube can be removed. The pins are turned daily until the lower jaw has reached a normal or even slightly longer-than-normal length. Once the mandible has been stretched to the appropriate length, the pins can often be removed, and the device is left in place for a few months while the new bone heals. The child is then returned to the operating room, and the distractor device and all of the screws are removed through the same incision. The infant is under general anesthesia for this procedure.

Historically, before MDO was invented, infants with severe PRS underwent a tracheostomy procedure. This involved a surgery in which a small incision was made in the midline of the neck directly into the trachea. A small plastic pipe was inserted through which air passed directly to the lungs, bypassing the child's mouth and the tongue blockage. Oxygen moved freely into and out of the lungs through the tube. A tracheostomy may be a life-saving procedure; however, it is a difficult burden for patients and families. It is reserved for patients with severe conditions that cannot be treated with any of the options discussed previously. For infants who have other congenital differences and cannot breathe well on their own, a tracheotomy is the preferred option. Often, unassisted breathing and feeding are unlikely for these children because of their syndromes or brain differences. Not every medical center has surgeons who perform MDO surgery, and tracheotomy is often the only option. These children are candidates for MDO surgery at a later time. If the procedure is successful, the tracheotomy tube is removed. Conversely, in patients who have undergone MDO surgery and still are unable to breathe well, a tracheotomy may be the only option to protect their airway from aspiration and lack of oxygen.

CONCLUSION

PRS can be a life-threatening condition that affects the breathing, eating, and growth of a newborn. However, with a team of specially trained care providers, children with PRS can receive the needed assessment, evaluation, and treatment required to successfully address these problems.

17

Sleep Apnea in Children With Cleft Lip and Palate

Jodi Gustave, Mark Splaingard

KEY POINTS

o Children with cleft lip and/or palate may have sleep-disordered breathing ranging from uncomplicated snoring to severe obstructive sleep apnea (OSA) with nocturnal oxygen *desaturation* and hypoventilation.

o Children with cleft lip and/or palate can develop sleep-disordered breathing after surgical procedures to improve speech or swallowing function.

o To recognize the connection between cleft lip and/or palate and sleep-disordered breathing, the anatomic and physiologic properties of the upper airway need to be understood. Multiple studies have documented the potential risk of sleep-disordered breathing in children with cleft lip and/or palate and after repairs.

o The best test to detect sleep-disordered breathing is an overnight *polysomnogram*, which is performed during a *sleep study*.

o Treatment of sleep-disordered breathing can include a variety of surgical procedures, but *continuous positive airway pressure* (CPAP) therapy may offer an excellent noninvasive option for some patients.

Sleep apnea (difficulty breathing during sleep) is a common problem in otherwise healthy children and adults. It is even more common in children and adults who have medical problems. Sleep apnea is seen more frequently in children with cleft lip and/or palate. Parents and caregivers should know what sleep apnea is, what signs to look for that indicate their child might have sleep apnea, what problems sleep apnea can cause, and what options exist to treat it.

WHAT IS A BREATHING PROBLEM DURING SLEEP?

Normal Breathing During Sleep

In all people, breathing gets a little bit worse during sleep. While we sleep, we take breaths that are a little more shallow. The depth of breathing is called the *tidal volume.* We also breathe a little faster. The speed of breathing is called the respiratory rate. For most people, this normal change in breathing pattern is not bad enough to cause problems, and they remain healthy.

When we fall asleep, our brain waves change shape. The waves are measured by a test called an electroencephalogram. Doctors use this information to know when we are asleep. The pattern and shapes of the brain waves seen during sleep have been given different names. There are two basic types of sleep, and each has its own brain wave pattern on an electroencephalogram. Rapid eye movement sleep is called *REM sleep,* and nonrapid eye movement sleep is called non-REM sleep. Non-REM sleep occurs when a person first falls asleep. It makes up about 70% to 80% of the total sleep time. There are three different types of non-REM sleep, which are called stage 1, stage 2, and stage 3. Stage 1 sleep usually occurs when we first fall asleep and lasts only a few minutes. Stage 2 sleep usually lasts about 50% of the total sleep time. Stage 3 sleep usually lasts about 25% of the total sleep time.

Breathing patterns and speed change during sleep, depending on the sleep stage. In stage 1 sleep, which occurs when a person first falls asleep, breathing becomes more irregular and starts to slow down. In stage 2 and stage 3 sleep, breathing becomes progressively more shallow (less air is taken in with each breath), but breathing is slightly faster.

REM sleep is very different from non-REM sleep. A person's brain waves on an electroencephalogram look similar to the brain waves seen when the person is awake. The eyes start to flutter, and many muscles become temporarily paralyzed. REM sleep is the time when dreams usually occur. Breathing is the worst during REM sleep; it is more irregular and more shallow, and the respiratory rate is faster than during any other sleep stage. This can cause a drop in blood oxygen levels, known as pO_2. Generally, any breathing problem a person has will become worse at night during REM sleep. Body positioning during sleep can also affect breathing during sleep. Lying on the back is called supine positioning. Breathing is generally the worst during REM sleep and when the child is lying in a supine position. This is called REM supine sleep.

During the night, a person typically cycles through the different sleep stages (stage 1, stage 2, stage 3, and REM). We move through all four stages every 60 to 90 minutes. This is known as a sleep cycle. The cycle repeats, usually four to six times throughout the night, with a different amount of time in each stage with each cycle. Generally, the cycles earlier in the night have more stage 3 sleep, and the cycles later in the night (from 5 to 8 AM) have more REM sleep. Therefore breathing at night will be the worst at the end of the sleep time, when more REM sleep occurs.

Sleep-Disordered Breathing and Sleep Apnea

Sleep-disordered breathing is a term used to describe the different types of breathing problems that occur only during sleep. These problems can be caused by many different conditions. The most common is asthma (wheezing and coughing that worsens during sleep). These breathing problems can affect how well a child sleeps and whether he or she is well rested the next day.

Sleep apnea is another very common cause of sleep-disordered breathing. Apnea is a lack of air movement from the nose and mouth into the lungs. There are two main types of apnea. One type is called *central sleep apnea,* in which the brain does not signal the muscles of breathing at the appropriate times. Children with central sleep apnea either have a very slow respiratory rate for their age, or they have very shallow movements of their chest wall during breathing efforts. This is a rare problem in children with a cleft lip and palate and usually only occurs in infancy, during some types of infections, or initially after surgery.

The second and most common type of sleep apnea in children is obstructive sleep apnea, or OSA. Children with this condition have a lack of air movement from the nose and mouth into the lungs, despite attempts to breathe, because of a blockage along this pathway (Fig. 17-1). The blockage might be in the nose, the mouth, or

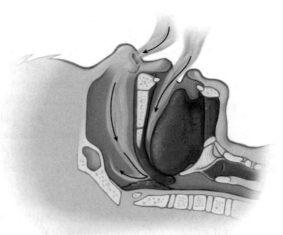

Fig. 17-1   Areas of blockage in apneic breathing.

the throat. These children may breathe well when they are awake, but when they fall asleep, breathing becomes more labored, with bigger chest movements and usually snoring (noise production that occurs when a child breathes in during sleep). These children may wake up periodically throughout the night because of blockage in their breathing. OSA can be a severe problem.

The severity of sleep apnea is scored by how many times a child either stops breathing (central sleep apnea) or has a blockage in breathing during every hour of sleep. This is called the *apnea-hypopnea index.* Children with mild OSA have one and a half to five obstructions per hour of sleep. Children with moderate OSA have five to ten obstructions per hour. Children with severe OSA have more than ten obstructions per hour.

HOW COMMON IS OBSTRUCTIVE SLEEP APNEA IN CHILDREN?

OSA can occur in infants and very young children. It is estimated that it occurs in about 2% to 3% of otherwise normal 5-year-old children. Approximately 10% of 5-year-old children snore more than three nights a week, and approximately one of four children who often snore actually have OSA that needs treatment. OSA is more common in children with enlarged *adenoids* and *tonsils,* obesity (excessive body weight), neurologic problems such as cerebral palsy, and craniofacial problems such as cleft lip and cleft palate.

Obstructive Sleep Apnea in Children With Cleft Lip and/or Cleft Palate

Infants and children with cleft lip and/or palate can have sleep-disordered breathing. About 10% of these children will be diagnosed with OSA based on a sleep study. This means that a child with cleft lip and/or cleft palate has approximately a three times greater chance of having sleep apnea than a child without a cleft. The highest risk of OSA is in children with cleft lip and/or palate from infancy to 2 years of age. In children with syndromes that include a cleft palate, such as those associated with *Pierre Robin sequence,* the chance of having OSA is even higher. Some authors report that up to 70% of children with Pierre Robin sequence have breathing problems during sleep.

WHY DO CHILDREN WITH CLEFT LIP AND PALATE HAVE MORE BREATHING PROBLEMS?

How the Facial Structure Affects Sleep

The shape and size of the face can affect how easy it is to take in air. A flattened face, blocked nose, small jaw, big tongue, and short neck can block airflow and make it harder to take in enough air during sleep. The palate is the roof of the mouth. Having a narrow palate or a high, arched palate can reduce the size of the airway and the amount of air that can be taken into the lungs during a breath. A reduction of the air that is taken in during each breath is called hypoventilation.

Breathing problems that take place during sleep and are caused by facial shape and size often occur in children with craniofacial differences, including cleft lip and/or cleft palate, Pierre Robin sequence, *Goldenhaar syndrome,* Treacher Collins syndrome, and velocardiofacial syndrome. Cleft lip and palate is the most common of these problems. One third of the children with cleft lip and/or palate have other physical abnormalities. They can have OSA because of their inability to take in enough air with each breath during sleep. These children can develop symptoms such as snoring, gasping (deep breaths followed by pauses), arching of the neck and head (neck hyperextension), and the inability to lie flat during sleep, preferring to sleep sitting up or while being held. They can develop these symptoms during sleep after surgeries to improve their speech, such as a posterior *pharyngeal flap* surgery.

Infants with Pierre Robin sequence have a cleft palate and a small chin, which is called *micrognathia* (Fig. 17-2). These infants can have severe problems with airway obstruction even when they are awake, but it usually becomes much worse during sleep. The tongue can fall back or get caught in the cleft of the palate, causing severe

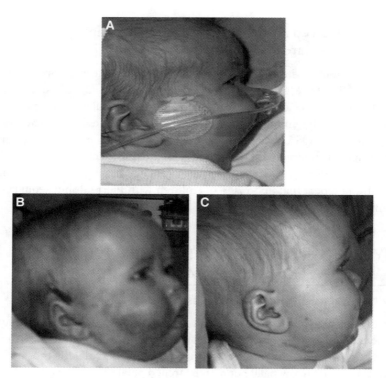

Fig. 17-2 Infant with Pierre Robin sequence. **A,** At birth. **B,** After surgery to lengthen the jaw. **C,** At 3 months of age.

breathing problems with very rapid breathing rates and obvious difficulty breathing, especially when the child is lying flat on the back. Surgeries are frequently necessary to help the child breathe normally during sleep.

WHY DOES SLEEP-DISORDERED BREATHING NEED TO BE TREATED?

Proper diagnosis and treatment of OSA are essential in children with cleft lip and palate. Untreated OSA has been proven to lead to many physical, behavioral, and learning problems. These include restless sleep, frequent awakening at night, failure to gain weight and grow properly, bed-wetting in children older than 6 years of age, hyperactivity, inattention, excessive daytime sleepiness, learning problems at school, high blood pressure, and if left untreated for a long time, heart failure and death.

HOW ARE BREATHING PROBLEMS DURING SLEEP DIAGNOSED IN CHILDREN?

Diagnosing Obstructive Sleep Apnea in Children With Cleft Lip and/or Palate

Children with cleft lip and/or palate are diagnosed with sleep apnea the same way as in other children. The adult caring for the child is usually the first to notice problems in the child's breathing that occur only at night. Symptoms of OSA include snoring, gasping, noisy breathing during sleep, sleeping in unusual positions such as sitting up or with the neck hyperextended, and waking up frequently at night. Family members might notice that occasionally the child stops breathing while sleeping. This is called apnea and is described as absent airflow that lasts longer than the time it takes for two regular breaths or 10 seconds, depending on the child's age. If a child has been potty trained and dry at night for longer than 3 months and starts wetting the bed again and snoring, OSA should be strongly suspected. Symptoms of OSA seen during the day include increased daytime sleepiness (a child older than 5 years of age starts taking afternoon naps again), hyperactivity, inattention, and learning problems.

The doctor may want to perform a couple of blood tests, including checking the hemoglobin or *serum bicarbonate* level. If these are abnormally high, OSA might be the cause. The doctor may ask the parents to observe or videotape their child during asleep. It is helpful to see and listen to the child's breathing at night. The best time to videotape is at approximately 6 AM when the child is most likely to be in REM sleep. Cyanosis (blue color of the child's skin caused by a low blood oxygen level) is not usually noted by parents, because the lights are generally off in the child's bedroom at night. An overnight continuous fingertip monitor called a pulse oximeter can be used in the home to detect low blood oxygen levels during the child's sleep, but low blood oxygen saturation is only seen in some children with severe OSA. Normal pulse oximetry results are seen in many children who have OSA, even those with severe OSA. Therefore pulse oximetry is not a good test to prove that a child does not have OSA. If the pulse oximeter result is abnormal, OSA should be strongly suspected and treated. However, a normal pulse oximetry study does not mean the child does not have OSA that requires treatment.

The test that is most useful in diagnosing sleep apnea is called a polysomnogram. This is also called a sleep study. During a sleep study, the child usually spends the night from about 7 PM until about 6 AM in a sleep laboratory in a hospital or outpatient facility. A parent is allowed to come with the child and sleep in a nearby bed. Infants younger than 4 months of age can have sleep studies during the daytime, because they sleep a lot during the daytime hours.

This is not a painful study. Small leads are pasted temporarily on the child's head for an electroencephalogram. This helps the doctor understand what stage of sleep the child is in. Small sensors are placed near the child's nose and mouth to measure airflow. This helps to understand when apnea occurs. Soft belts are placed over the child's chest and abdomen to help determine whether movements of the chest or stomach occur at the same time as the apnea. This helps the doctors decide whether the child is having central or obstructive apneas during sleep. The heart rate is measured by electrocardiogram leads. Blood oxygen levels are measured with pulse oximetry, in which a small sensor is placed on the finger or heel. All of this information is collected continuously and displayed on a computer screen while the child is sleeping. After the study, a sleep technician will spend a couple of hours looking at each 30-second period of sleep and organizing the different sleep stages and breathing patterns recorded. Then, a doctor trained in sleep medicine reviews all of the data and makes a diagnosis. A sleep study helps to gather other information about the patient's sleep as well.

HOW ARE BREATHING PROBLEMS DURING SLEEP TREATED?

Treatments for Children Without Clefts Who Have Obstructive Sleep Apnea

Children without clefts who are 2 to 8 years of age often develop OSA. This is usually caused by large tonsils, large adenoids, or obesity. Treatment of OSA at these ages can include *tonsillectomy* (the removal of the tonsils, which are large pieces of *lymphoid tissue* behind the tongue) and/or *adenoidectomy* (the removal of the adenoids, which are large pieces of lymphoid tissue at the back of the nose and above the palate). These two surgical procedures are the second most common surgical procedures performed during childhood and help most children breathe more easily and efficiently during sleep.

Sometimes OSA is so severe in a child without a cleft that it is not completely corrected by surgery. A child with mild or moderate OSA after adenoidectomy or tonsillectomy can be treated with positional therapy. This involves having the child sleep lying on the stomach (prone positioning) or with the head elevated with pillows or a wedge.

Children with more severe OSA can be treated with a CPAP device (Fig. 17-3). This treatment can be continued for a long time, until the OSA improves with weight loss or further facial growth. CPAP is a therapy that uses a machine to blow air gently into the child's nose through a nasal mask or prongs or into both the nose

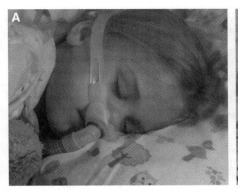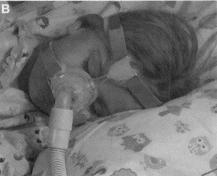

Fig. 17-3 Pediatric CPAP masks. **A,** Nasal mask. **B,** Full-face mask.

and mouth using a full-face mask. The amount of air pressure that is required to open the child's airway is determined during an overnight sleep study while the child is wearing the mask. This sleep study is called a *CPAP titration study.* The success of CPAP treatment for OSA depends on the cooperation of the child (how well the child can wear the mask throughout the period of sleep), how much improvement is expected as the child grows, and the social support available for the child. The ability to successfully wear a CPAP mask throughout the night to treat OSA is called CPAP compliance and generally is about 50% in children. A small number of children without cleft may require more surgeries to improve OSA.

Treatment of Obstructive Sleep Apnea in Children With Cleft Lip and/or Palate

After the initial cleft lip and palate repairs during the first year of life, some children develop OSA between 2 and 8 years of age. Some children with cleft lip and palate can develop problems with speech or swallowing (liquids come out of the nose). They require surgery such as a pharyngeal flap after the palate repair. Although OSA might be present before these surgeries, it is a possible negative effect of these procedures.

Treatment of children with cleft lip and/or palate who have OSA depends on the severity of the OSA. If OSA is mild, positional treatment during sleep may be all that is needed. These children should avoid sleeping on their back. The best positions are generally a semisitting position or a prone position. This can become difficult once the child gets bigger and is able to change positions without help. Treatment of OSA in these children can include tonsillectomy and/or adenoidectomy. However, these procedures can be more complicated in a child with a repaired cleft lip and palate than in a child without a cleft because of swallowing and speech concerns. A decision is usually made by both the plastic surgeon and the ear, nose, and throat surgeon.

Children with repaired cleft lip and palate who are at least 2 years old and have more severe OSA can be treated temporarily with CPAP. This has become possible only in the past 15 years, ever since small pediatric masks that can fit a child's nose have become available. This treatment can be continued for a long time, until the OSA improves with further facial growth and development. CPAP may also be a good treatment option for children who develop OSA after speech surgery that is expected to improve in a few months.

Children with the most severe OSA who either cannot tolerate CPAP or who do not have OSA that is corrected by CPAP may require additional surgeries. One type of surgery is called a tracheostomy. In this procedure, a hole is created in the windpipe through the front of the neck, and a tube is inserted. The tube is called a tracheostomy tube. The child can breathe through the tracheostomy tube during sleep. The tube bypasses the blocked area that prevents air from flowing upward from the lungs and into the throat, mouth, and nose. With newer surgeries, a tracheostomy is not required as often as it was 15 years ago. A tracheostomy may be necessary to treat severe OSA until further craniofacial surgery can be performed when the child is older.

CONCLUSION

Children with a cleft lip and cleft palate are at risk of developing OSA. Snoring, gasping at night, and pauses in breathing are the major signs of OSA. A sleep study is the best way to diagnose the presence of OSA and its severity. Treatments for sleep apnea include surgery, special positioning, and CPAP therapy.

Part V

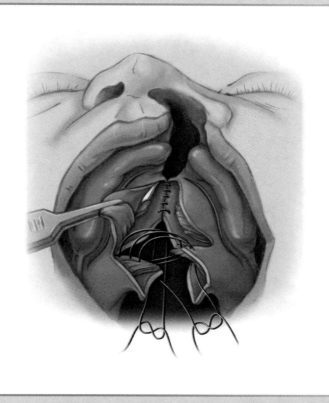

Cleft Lip and Palate Repair

18

Anesthesia for Cleft Patients

E. Gail Shaffer, Franklyn P. Cladis

KEY POINTS

○ Anesthesia is very safe for children and infants.

○ Many specific steps are taken before, during, and after surgery to make sure the child is safe and comfortable.

○ Nausea and vomiting are the most common side effects of anesthesia.

Several hundred years ago, patients who had cleft lip and palate surgery were not given an anesthetic or pain medication. Today, anesthesia is always provided for this procedure, making the surgery much safer. For parents, this can be the most concerning part of the surgery. The good news is that anesthesia for infants and children is extremely safe. We hope this chapter provides information that will help to make the day of surgery less stressful. It will focus on what parents can expect before, during, and after the surgery with regard to anesthesia.

BEFORE THE SURGERY

Cleft lip and palate surgery is usually performed when the patient is young. The surgeon will determine the best age and time of surgery for each patient. Most commonly, a cleft lip is repaired when the child is 3 to 6 months of age, and a cleft palate is repaired when the child is age 9 to 18 months of age. Other surgeries on the mouth may be needed as the child gets older.

Type of Food or Liquid	Duration of Fast Before Surgery (hours)
Clear liquids (water, white grape juice, or apple juice without pulp)	2
Breast milk	4
Formula (may include cow's milk if the infant is younger than 6 to 12 months)	6
Food (including cow's milk)	8

Table 18-1 Fasting Guidelines for Surgery

Some children with cleft lip and palate are completely healthy. However, others have trouble swallowing and feeding and may be malnourished. Some children have many medical concerns, including conditions of the heart, brain and nervous system, or muscle and bone. Parents of children who have several medical issues in addition to a cleft lip and/or palate might be asked to come to the hospital for a meeting with the anesthesia team before the day of surgery. If the child is otherwise healthy, this meeting may not be needed until the day of surgery. Before the day of surgery, parents are given instructions about giving medications, food, and drinks in preparation of surgery, along with other essential information. It is very important to follow these instructions. Patients undergoing anesthesia are asked to fast for a period of time before the surgery. This ensures that the stomach is empty and decreases the risk of stomach contents entering the lungs during anesthesia (aspiration). Typical fasting times are provided in Table 18-1; however, the parents should follow the directions provided by their specific anesthesia team, who will provide the anesthetic to the child.

THE DAY OF SURGERY

Most children will come to the hospital on the morning of the surgery, unless they have already been hospitalized for another reason. It is no longer common for children to come to the hospital the night before surgery.

After checking in, the parents and their child will be taken to an area to prepare for surgery (sometimes called the preoperative area). There, parents will be asked many questions about the child's medical conditions, medications, allergies, previous surgeries, family history, and most recent meal. If the child has had a significant cold in the past 2 weeks, the anesthesia team will want to know about this. The safest time to have anesthesia is at least 2 weeks after a cold. If the child arrives for elective surgery with a significant cold (fever, yellow drainage from the nose, a bad cough, and obviously sick), surgery might be postponed for 2 weeks for safety. The anesthesiologist will ask about any family history of anesthesia-related complications, because some of these may be genetic. For example, *malignant hyperthermia* is a very rare and serious reaction to anesthesia that is characterized by high fever, redness, and muscle rigidity. If anyone in the family has had this type of reaction to anesthesia, this information needs to be shared with the anesthesia team. There are methods of providing anesthesia that can prevent this type of anesthesia-related problem.

The anesthesia team will discuss the method of anesthesia with the parents before surgery. The child may be given a sedative medication called midazolam (Versed is another name). This can be taken by mouth or placed in the nose like nose drops. This medication is very safe and effective. However, in a small number of children, it can have the opposite effect and make them hyperactive. In addition to sedating the child, the medication will help with possible separation anxiety, which can be upsetting to both the child and the parent. Patients younger than 10 months typically do not need this medication.

When it is time to go to surgery, the child will be taken by the anesthesia team to the operating room. Some hospitals let the parents stay with their child while he or she is sedated and anesthetized (falls asleep under anesthesia). This will be discussed with the parents before surgery. An anesthesia gas can be given through a mask, or a medication can be given through an intravenous (IV) line. The mask might be flavored to make it more pleasant.

DURING THE SURGERY

Parents who are allowed to be in the operating room or a nearby room while their child goes to sleep will then be taken to the waiting area. After the child is asleep, an IV line will be placed, usually in the hand, arm, or foot. Sometimes two IV lines are needed. Next, a breathing tube will be placed in the windpipe (trachea) to protect the lungs during surgery. This will be taped to the cheeks to keep it in place. The tape occasionally causes redness on the cheeks after surgery, but this usually goes away quickly.

During the entire surgery, the child will be asleep, because the anesthesia team will continue to give anesthesia gas and IV medications. They might also give pain medication, nausea medication, an antibiotic, and medicine to reduce swelling (a steroid).

At the end of surgery, the anesthesiologist will make certain that the child is breathing well and does not have too much swelling in the mouth. The breathing tube will be removed when it is safe to do so. Oxygen will be given through a mask placed on the child's face to help with breathing. Some patients require a small tube to be placed in the nose (nasopharyngeal airway) to help with breathing after the surgery.

AFTER THE SURGERY

Immediately after the surgery is finished, many children will go to a recovery area to wake up. A small number of children may need to go to an intensive care unit (ICU) after surgery. In the recovery room, a nurse will make sure that the child is breathing well, has a normal blood pressure and heart rate, and is comfortable. The child will still have an IV line in place and may receive IV fluids, pain medication, or nausea medication. Some children will be very sedated, and some will be more awake. Parents are brought to see their child when he or she is fully awake. The surgeon will give instructions to the parents about when their child can begin to eat and drink. Some children wake up from anesthesia very upset. This is probably related to a combination of discomfort from the surgery, disorientation from the anesthesia, hunger, and fear. A phenomenon called emergence delirium can occur, which is characterized by extreme irritability, combativeness, and inconsolability. It occurs in approximately 10% to 15% of pediatric patients. It is important during this time to prevent patients from hurting themselves (for example, by falling out of bed and hitting their head). This upsetting process settles down and goes away within 15 minutes in almost all patients. The anesthesiologist may give an additional sedative to help the child calm down more quickly.

PAIN MANAGEMENT

Pain relief during and after the child's surgery is very important. The anesthesiologist can give a variety of different medications for pain relief. During the surgery, these medications will likely be given through the IV line, or as a suppository. When the child is awake in the recovery room, pain medication can be given through the IV line or by mouth. The goal of the pain medication is to make the child comfortable without unpleasant side effects. Side effects of opioid-based pain medications (for example, morphine, hydromorphone, and oxycodone) can include itching, nausea and vomiting, and problems with breathing. For these reasons, the anesthesiologist will often give several different types of medication to minimize side effects. Nonopioid pain medications include acetaminophen (Tylenol) and nonsteroidal antiinflammatories (NSAIDs) such as ibuprofen or ketorolac. Some surgeons do not allow ibuprofen or ketorolac to be given, because they think that these medications can increase the risk of bleeding.

In addition to IV pain medications, anesthesiologists or surgeons can give the child a nerve block for pain relief. A nerve block is an injection of a numbing medication (similar to the medicine that the dentist injects in the mouth) that can make the lip area numb so the child does not feel pain for several hours. A nerve block may be given while the child is under anesthesia so that he or she will not feel or remember it.

RECOVERY

Most infants and children do very well after anesthesia and surgery and have no residual effects. Nausea and vomiting are the most common negative effects of anesthesia. Nausea is more likely to occur in patients 3 years of age or older, after surgery that lasts longer than 30 minutes, and in patients who have a personal or family history of nausea and vomiting after surgery. The good news is that most children having cleft lip and palate surgery are younger than 3 years of age and have a smaller risk of nausea and vomiting. Some children have subtle behavioral changes for up to 2 weeks after undergoing anesthesia and surgery. These changes include an increase in tantrums, bed-wetting, and separation anxiety. These behaviors resolve during the first 2 weeks after surgery in 80% of children. In general, these are subtle changes that do not cause long-lasting issues.

CONCLUSION

Today, children undergoing cleft lip and palate surgery benefit from advanced anesthesia techniques that are safe and effective. After consideration of the child's unique health picture and surgical needs, the anesthesiologist will design an anesthesia treatment plan. Side effects of anesthesia are rare and tend to resolve very quickly after surgery. The most common side effects are nausea and vomiting. A specially trained team led by an anesthesiologist ensures that children having surgery are safe and comfortable before, during, and after the procedure.

19

Cleft Lip and Nose Adhesion

Oluwaseun A. Adetayo, Richard E. Kirschner, Joseph E. Losee

KEY POINTS

- A *cleft lip and nose adhesion* is an alternative to presurgical infant orthopedic procedures that helps to prepare the cleft lip for the final repair.

- The disadvantages and risks of a cleft lip and nose adhesion are usually minimal.

- The treatment plan is individualized for each baby.

- Parents need to discuss postoperative care with their baby's doctors.

A cleft lip and nose adhesion is a procedure that is sometimes performed as part of a child's cleft care. Not all children with a cleft require this procedure. However, when a cleft lip and nose adhesion is performed, it is the first of two stages. It prepares the cleft for the second stage, which is the actual (definitive) cleft lip repair used to surgically repair the lip and nose. A cleft lip and nose adhesion helps to narrow the width of the baby's cleft to facilitate the definitive lip repair by converting a "complete cleft" into an "incomplete cleft" (see Chapter 27).

In general, the lip adhesion procedure is done when the child is approximately 2 to 3 months of age. The definitive cleft lip and nose repair is performed when the child is approximately 4 to 6 months of age. However, some babies are seen when they are older. These children are also eligible for this procedure.

ADVANTAGES AND DISADVANTAGES

For families who cannot participate in *presurgical infant orthopedics* such as nasoalveolar molding (see Chapter 27), a cleft lip and nose adhesion can be a good alternative. It offers more convenience for families with travel, social, financial, and other constraints that prevent participation in the other preoperative treatments. A cleft lip and nose adhesion helps to align the lip and nose, shape the alveolus (gum ridge), and decrease the size of the gap between the cleft lip edges.

The disadvantages include an additional surgery, the potential anesthetic risk, and the possibility of wound separation and increased scar formation.

PREOPERATIVE CONSIDERATIONS

The surgeon will discuss the surgical procedure with the parents before the day of the surgery. The parents will have the opportunity to meet with the anesthesiologist and other members of the team who will care for their child.

OPERATIVE PROCEDURE

After the child is safely under a general anesthesia, small incisions are made on either side of the cleft lip, near the junction of the lip and the nose. Incisions are made just inside the mouth to release the lip on the side of the face and move it toward the middle. The lip and nose are partially sewn together (Figs. 19-1 and 19-2). Often a permanent stitch is placed inside the cheeks and lips to help keep the lips together while they heal; this stitch is taken out at the time of the definitive cleft lip and nose repair. Fig. 19-3, *A*, shows a child who was born with a right-sided complete cleft lip and nose who underwent a cleft lip and nose adhesion. Fig. 19-3, *B*, shows the child after the definitive repair of the cleft lip.

PATIENT EXAMPLES

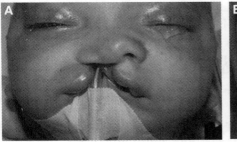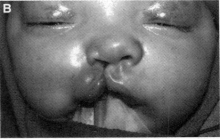

Fig. 19-1   A child with a right-sided unilateral cleft lip. **A,** Before cleft lip and nose adhesion. **B,** Immediately after cleft lip and nose adhesion.

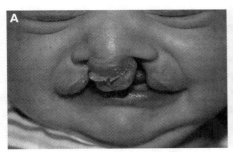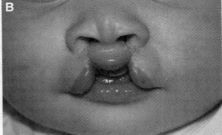

Fig. 19-2   A child with a bilateral complete cleft lip. **A,** Before cleft lip and nose adhesion. **B,** Several weeks after cleft lip and nose adhesion.

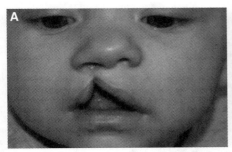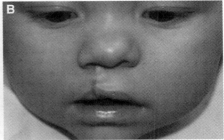

Fig. 19-3   A child born with a right-sided complete cleft lip. **A,** After cleft lip and nose adhesion. **B,** After definitive cleft lip and nose repair.

COMPLICATIONS

A cleft lip and nose adhesion is usually very safe, with few potential complications. One postoperative complication can be breakdown of the skin and separation of the adhesion. If the surgeon placed a permanent internal stitch (intended to be removed at the time of definitive cleft lip repair), this stitch often helps keep the edges of the lip together despite the breakdown of the skin. If this is the case, the effect of the cleft lip and nose adhesion is maintained.

In rare instances, breakdown of the skin may result in a complete loss of the adhesion, and the surgeon will discuss the options and alternatives at that time. Other potential complications include those common to most surgeries and include bleeding, infection, and bad scarring. These will be discussed at the preoperative visit.

POSTOPERATIVE CARE AND CONSIDERATIONS

After surgery, the child is usually monitored in the hospital overnight. Most patients go home the following day, provided they are recovering well. In general, no major changes are made to the feeding regimen, but the doctor will discuss any desired changes with the parents. Some doctors prefer to place baby arm splints/restraints to prevent injury to the surgery site on the lip and nose. This will be discussed with the parents. Parents may need to provide cleaning and hygiene care for the child's lip and nose after surgery. The doctor and his or her team will discuss their preferred routine and demonstrate how to perform the desired postoperative care regimen. Some surgeons will require the use of nasal stents or splints after surgery to help shape the nose (Fig. 19-4).

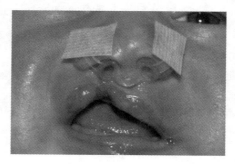

Fig. 19-4   A child with nasal stents (splints) in place after cleft lip and nose adhesion.

CONCLUSION

A cleft lip and nose adhesion is one of the different techniques that can be performed before, and help "set the stage" for, the definitive cleft lip and nose repair. When presurgical infant orthopedics are not an option for families, the cleft lip and nose adhesion procedure is a powerful tool to prepare a child for definitive cleft lip and nose surgery.

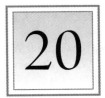

20

Unilateral Cleft Lip and Nose Repair

Ashley Salyer, Adelle Green, Kenneth E. Salyer

KEY POINTS

○ Cleft lip of any severity can be treated successfully.

○ Early, complete evaluation by an experienced team is important.

○ Repair of the lip and nose is essential for normal appearance, function, and growth.

○ The protocol for cleft lip repair varies from center to center. It may be performed in one or two stages. Some centers recommend lip taping, nasoalveolar molding, or another form of presurgical orthopedics before lip repair.

Every parent of a newborn baby with a cleft lip and palate should understand that with state-of-the-art treatment by an experienced multidisciplinary or interdisciplinary team, the child will be able enjoy a good quality of life and reach his or her full potential. Over time, many visits to the team and to multiple care providers will be necessary. In addition, a number of surgical procedures will be needed. These will be coordinated with speech therapy, orthodontics, and other treatment. The goal of team care is to achieve the best possible appearance and normal speech to promote acceptance by the child's peers.

Parents of a newborn baby with a cleft will encounter many challenges. One of the first challenges is to ensure successful feeding using the special bottles, nipples, and techniques that are available (see Chapter 7 for a discussion of this topic). The next major challenge is surgery. When surgery is performed by an experienced surgeon and supported by a qualified team, excellent outcomes can be expected. A child with a complete cleft of the lip and palate is likely to undergo at least five operations by the time he or she is fully grown. The surgical plan usually includes one or two procedures to repair the lip and nose and another to repair the palate, all during infancy. Later, when the child is approximately 7 to 8 years of age, an orthodontist will determine when eruption of the adult teeth into the cleft area is soon to begin. At this time, if the alveolus or gum ridge is clefted and missing necessary bone, alveolar bone grafting is performed to create a solid dental arch and to allow the teeth to erupt.

Every cleft-affected child should have a complete team evaluation early in life. The team is likely to include many different specialists (see Chapter 1). Ultimately, the care provided by the team's surgeon will play perhaps the greatest role in determining the quality of outcomes. This chapter discusses the primary surgery of the lip and nose and necessary supportive care.

PREOPERATIVE CONSIDERATIONS

Timing

Some parents request that the cleft be repaired immediately after birth. However, this type of surgery on the newborn at such an early age can carry a higher risk and may result in a poor-quality repair. Therefore most cleft lip and palate treatment centers prefer to wait to perform the initial lip repair until the child is approximately 3 months of age.

There are several reasons for this delay. First, a healthy, vigorous child weighing more than 10 pounds is better able to tolerate the anesthesia and surgery. Second, the waiting period allows ample time to thoroughly diagnose the extent and characteristics of the cleft and any additional or associated problems that might be present. Waiting allows time to adequately plan immediate and long-term treatment. Finally, the facial structures of a child of 3 months of age are significantly larger than those of a newborn; this facilitates the technical aspects of the surgery, resulting in a much better aesthetic and functional outcome.

Preoperative Treatment

In some centers, a preliminary lip adhesion may be performed before the definitive lip repair. A lip adhesion is a partial repair of the lip that facilitates narrowing of the cleft and remodeling of the lip and nose (see Chapter 19). Many centers recommend the use of a nonsurgical technique known as *presurgical infant orthopedics* to prepare the patient for surgical repair (see Chapter 27). This often involves lip taping or the use of special appliances to guide the two sides of the cleft palate into a more favorable position. Nasoalveolar molding involves the use of appliances to reshape the nose before the surgical repair. The surgeon and orthodontist on the team should discuss their preferences for presurgical management with each family, providing information about the potential benefits of each protocol and the associated investment of time, effort, and cost.

Primary Repair

Primary repair of the cleft lip and nose is generally performed when the child is 3 to 6 months of age. This first operation is very important, creating the foundation for future care and outcomes. An experienced cleft surgeon with the support of an interdisciplinary team should perform the procedure.

A child's general health is very important in determining his or her readiness for surgery. This is why a complete assessment by the team is essential. All associated anomalies or medical problems need to be recognized and treated before lip repair surgery is performed.

The otolaryngologist on the team will perform a preoperative assessment to determine whether the child has fluid behind the eardrum. If fluid is present, insertion of tubes in the eardrum may be indicated at the time of lip repair or later (see Chapter 14). The need for and timing of ear tube placement depends on the judgment and experience of the otolaryngologist and the surgical protocol used by the team.

OPERATIVE PROCEDURES

Repair of the Unilateral Cleft Lip and Nose: Philosophy

Every child with a unilateral cleft of the lip presents a unique surgical challenge. In all cases, experienced surgeons provide the best results. Many techniques have been described for repair of a unilateral cleft lip, and most surgeons have a specific preference. All techniques involve making cuts within the tissues next to the cleft and rearranging them to repair the lip and restore lip and nasal tip symmetry. Tissue from elsewhere in the body is not added to the lip; all of the tissue necessary is present in the area of the cleft. Some surgeons place sutures that will dissolve on their own; others place sutures that need to be removed after the tissues heal.

Surgeons consider several key elements to obtain the best results after cleft lip repair. First, nasal involvement is nearly always present; therefore the nasal tip should be addressed to some degree at the time of primary lip surgery. The extent to which

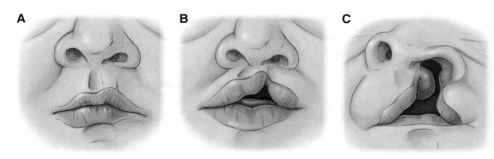

Fig. 20-1 Types of unilateral cleft lip. **A,** Microform. **B,** Incomplete. **C,** Complete.

the nasal cleft is corrected in infancy depends largely on the surgeon's preference. Some surgeons attempt a near-total correction of the nasal cleft at the time of lip repair, whereas others prefer to more completely address the nasal asymmetry later in childhood. Second, the cleft lip and nose is dynamic (changing) and needs to be treated throughout the child's growth and development. Therefore long-term treatment protocols rather than one-time surgical solutions should be the rule.

The severity of a unilateral cleft lip varies greatly (Fig. 20-1). Some children have minor notching at the lower border of the lip. This is referred to as a microform cleft lip. In others, the cleft extends higher into the lip, with a bridge of skin remaining beneath the nose. This is classified as an incomplete cleft lip. Finally, the cleft can extend through the entire lip and into the floor of the nose, a condition known as a complete cleft lip. In all cases, the cleft may or may not extend into the alveolus (gums) and the palate. When the cleft extends through the alveolus, alveolar bone grafting will be required later during childhood (see Chapter 29).

Operative Repair

Surgery is performed in the hospital or an outpatient surgical facility. The child is under general anesthesia during the operation. Admission procedures are completed on or before the day of surgery. Generally, a unilateral cleft lip and nose is repaired in approximately 1 to 3 hours. Children are discharged home once they are comfortable and feeding well. At some centers, children are discharged on the day of surgery; at others, an overnight stay is recommended.

Regardless of the technique used, the objective of surgery is to reconstruct the aesthetic and functional aspects of the lip and nose so that they will look and function as normally as possible. Incisions will be made that allow the tissues to be rearranged to achieve excellent lip contour and symmetry (Fig. 20-2). In both complete and incomplete clefts, the muscle that allows normal motion and func-

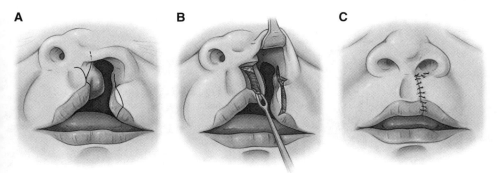

Fig. 20-2   Unilateral cleft lip repair. **A,** Design. **B,** Dissection. **C,** Completed repair.

tion of the lip is disrupted. This muscle will be repaired at the time of the initial lip repair. The cleft nose is often treated at the same time as the primary lip repair, depending on the surgeon's preference. This is the single most important operation on the nose and lip, although additional surgery to achieve better nasal form may be performed when the child is older.

Technical precision at the time of the primary lip and nose operation is critical for an outstanding long-term outcome. The interdisciplinary team and surgeon should have extensive experience and be able to demonstrate excellent long-term outcomes. Parental compliance with team protocols, along with adherence to the preoperative and postoperative instructions, are also an important factor in ensuring the best outcome possible.

POSTOPERATIVE CARE

Infants may resume feeding after the lip repair once they have fully recovered from the anesthesia. Some surgeons allow infants to return to bottle- or breast-feeding immediately, whereas others prefer that they use cups or syringes.

Some surgeons prescribe the use of arm splints after surgery. These arm restraints help protect the lip and nose repair by keeping the child's fingers away from the fresh surgical site. The parents will need to clean encrusted fluid and blood from the lip incision. The care team will demonstrate the best technique before the child is discharged from the hospital.

Some surgeons place a silicone stent into the nose at the completion of the surgical repair to maintain symmetry of the nasal tip (Figs. 20-3 through 20-5). The stent is maintained for 3 to 6 months; parents will be instructed on how to clean it daily.

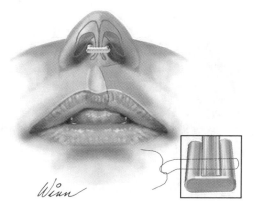

Fig. 20-3 Placement of a postoperative silicone nasal stent.

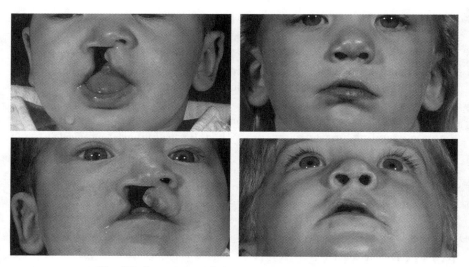

Fig. 20-4 Patient with a complete right-sided cleft lip.

Depending on the type of suture placed to close the lip and nose incisions, some will need to be removed several days after surgery. Parents should ensure that they fully understand and comply with the care prescribed by their team.

COMPLICATIONS

Cleft lip and nasal repair in healthy infants is generally a very safe procedure. Major complications after surgery are uncommon.

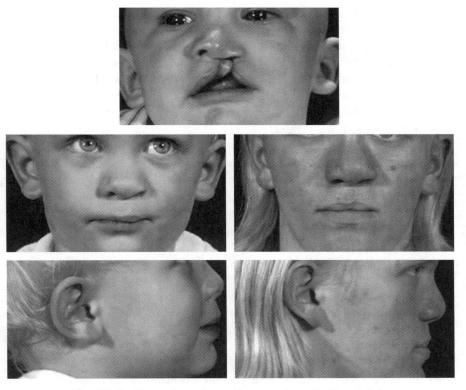

Fig. 20-5   Series of a patient with a complete left-sided cleft lip.

Anesthesia

When anesthesia is given by experienced pediatric anesthesiologists, complications from primary cleft repairs are extremely unusual. Side effects (such as nausea or vomiting) or adverse reactions (such as a rash) that result from anesthesia can occur, as with any medication, but they are rare. Parents will be asked to provide the anesthesiologist with a medical history of both their child and their family members to ensure that the anesthesia is as safe as possible for their child (see Chapter 18).

Wound Healing

Wound healing is uncomplicated in almost all cleft repairs. If the lip is closed under extreme tension, however, the incision can separate. This is called dehiscence and is rare. If this occurs, the lip will need to be rerepaired.

Scarring in the nose can occur in the nostril on the cleft side for many reasons. When scarring from surgery results in a small nostril, airflow through the nose can be decreased, and the desired aesthetic result is not achieved. Atypical scarring within the nostril can cause *vestibular stenosis* (narrowing of the nostril), which can be difficult to correct. In some cases it may be necessary to insert a nasal stent to prevent additional narrowing of the nostril. The stent may need to be worn for several months. Secondary surgical correction with tissue grafts or flaps can improve vestibular stenosis.

Scar maturation in infants may take a year or longer. During this time the scar may become pink and somewhat thickened and firm. With time, the appearance and texture of the scar will improve. Protocols for scar management vary widely, but scar massage is frequently prescribed to optimize scar maturation and appearance. Delicate surgical technique and compliance with postoperative instructions for scar management most often ensure satisfactory scar maturation and appearance. In some cases, however, a thick scar, referred to as a *hypertrophic scar,* persists and requires treatment. A hypertrophic scar can usually be managed effectively with pressure from taping and frequent massage. Rarely, injection of a corticosteroid preparation into the scar may be necessary.

Wound Infection

Infection in the lip or nose after primary repair is extremely uncommon. If it occurs, antibiotics will be given. Rarely, surgical drainage is required.

Bleeding

Bleeding after cleft lip repair is extremely rare and occurs most frequently in children with an undiagnosed blood condition that prevents normal clotting. Management of these patients requires consultation with a pediatric hematologist (a specialist in disorders of the blood) for proper evaluation and treatment.

CONCLUSION

Cleft lip repair is often the first surgical procedure in the journey of a cleft-affected infant. Parents can be overwhelmed. However, the guidance and support of an experienced cleft-craniofacial team can help to ease the process. Meticulous surgical technique and postoperative care generally result in very favorable functional and aesthetic outcomes.

21

Bilateral Cleft Lip and Nose Repair

Philip Kuo-Ting Chen

KEY POINTS

○ Good health is essential for children who have surgery to repair their cleft lip and nose.

○ Nasoalveolar molding and other forms of presurgical infant orthopedics can facilitate repair of the cleft lip and nose (see Chapter 27).

○ The immediate postoperative result will change over time.

○ The best outcomes in cleft lip and nose repair depend on cooperation between the patient, the family, and the cleft team.

Many parents are shocked the first time they see their cleft-affected child. This is especially true for parents of babies with bilateral cleft lips. A bilateral cleft lip is split into three parts, and the nose is distorted, wide, and flat. However, nonsurgical and surgical techniques can be performed to correct these differences.

Parents and surgeons have more treatment options today. In the 1980s, babies born with a bilateral cleft lip had more surgeries with less satisfactory outcomes, compared with those born with a unilateral cleft lip. Bilateral cleft lips were more difficult to repair. A technique called presurgical nasoalveolar molding was developed in the mid- to late 1990s to greatly improve the outcomes of bilateral cleft lip and nose repair (see Chapter 27). Before the child has surgery, the width of the cleft and the asymmetry of the upper jaw can be gradually improved with an orthodontic device. These preoperative adjustments can also improve the appearance of the nose and make the cleft lip surgery more straightforward. Now, babies born with a bilateral cleft lip have a similar number of surgeries and comparable outcomes to those with a unilateral cleft lip. At centers that do not offer nasoalveolar molding, other forms of presurgical infant orthopedics may be available.

PREOPERATIVE CONSIDERATIONS

Nasoalveolar molding has numerous benefits. It decreases the cleft width, lengthens the columella, and makes the upper jaw more symmetrical. The narrower the cleft, the more straightforward the surgical repair. A longer columella will improve the nasal shape after the repair. The molding procedure should start as early as possible. The desired result is usually achieved in approximately 2 to 3 months. The next procedure, surgery to close the cleft, will be performed when the child is 3 to 6 months of age. Infants with a cleft should be brought to the cleft clinic soon after birth. The orthodontist will take an impression of the upper jaw and make the nasoalveolar molding device. The device is made of an acrylic plate for the anterior part of the palatal cleft, with two extensions for the nose (Fig. 21-1). It helps the parents feed the baby. The parents will need to bring the child back to the cleft clinic every 1 to 2 weeks to have the device adjusted. The frequency of the visits and the cost of the treatment are the two primary drawbacks of nasoalveolar molding (Fig. 21- 2).

Babies should be in good health when they have surgery. Surgeons refer to a rule of 10 for lip repair: The child should be older than 10 weeks of age, the body weight should be more than 10 pounds, hemoglobin should be higher than 10 g/dl, and the white blood cell count should be less than 10,000/μl. The first three requirements

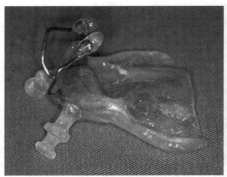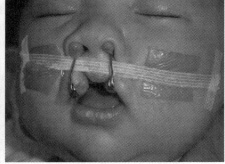

Fig. 21-1   Device for nasoalveolar molding.

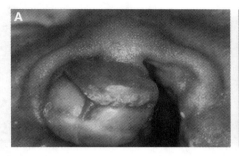
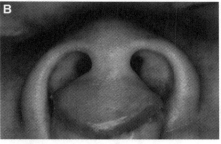

Fig. 21-2   This baby has a bilateral cleft lip and palate. **A,** The baby is seen at the initial visit. **B,** Nasoalveolar molding is completed. The upper lip and the length of the columella are improved.

ensure that the infant has reasonably good heart and lung function and is growing appropriately through good nutrition. The last requirement implies that the infant has no upper respiratory tract infections. Because the surgery will be performed while the child is under general anesthesia, good function of the heart and lungs and the absence of respiratory tract infections are important prerequisites. Good nutrition aids the healing process. If the child has any other systemic disease (for example, congenital heart disease), the surgeon and the anesthesiologist should be notified. Sometimes other specialists must be consulted to evaluate the possible risks from these conditions.

Some hospitals perform bilateral cleft lip and nose repair on an outpatient surgery basis, which means that the child will be discharged from the hospital soon after recovery from general anesthesia. However, most surgeons prefer that the patient stay in the hospital at least overnight.

Anesthesia requires a period of fasting before surgery called NPO time. NPO refers to the Latin words nihil per os, meaning nothing by mouth. The baby's stomach should be empty to prevent aspiration during the surgery. The length of fasting time depends on the child's age. The operating time varies from surgeon to surgeon.

OPERATIVE PROCEDURE

Several techniques are available to repair a bilateral cleft lip. The goal of the surgery is to achieve a balanced-looking lip and nose. This is somewhat difficult, because the lip and nose are always asymmetrical, even after nasoalveolar molding is

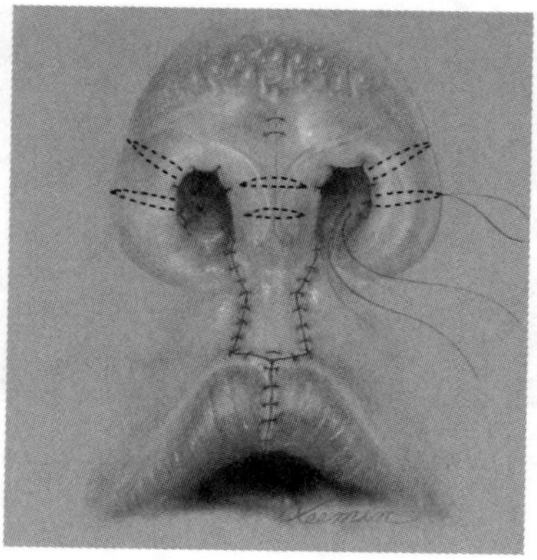

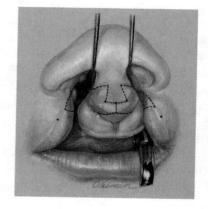

Fig. 21-3   Closing the lip in layers.

Fig. 21-4   Marking incisions for nose repair.

completed. The bony gaps are also asymmetrical. The surgeons will try their best to achieve symmetry by shortening or lengthening different parts of the tissues.

The lip is closed in layers. The inside skin or mucosa is closed as well as the muscle of the lip and then the skin of the lip. Skin from the *prolabium* (the middle third piece of the unrepaired upper lip) is used to make the *philtrum* (the central part of the repaired lip) (Fig. 21-3). Most surgeons operate on the nose at the time of the lip surgery. Many accomplish this with incisions on the nose to gain access to the cartilage in the tip of the nose (Fig. 21-4).

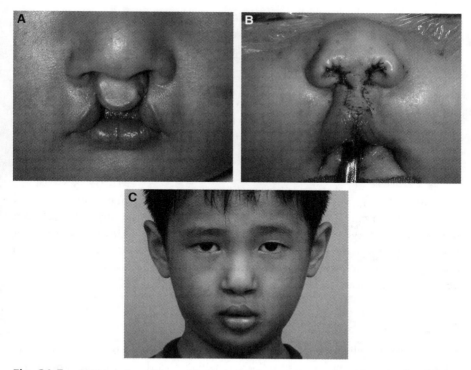

Fig. 21-5   A, This baby will have bilateral cleft lip and nose surgery. **B,** Immediately after surgery, the lip and nose have a tight and strange appearance. **C,** The child is seen 7 years after surgery.

The lip may look tight and strange immediately after surgery, because the tissue is deficient and the surgeon needs to pull the separated parts together (Fig. 21-5, *A*). However, the tissue will stretch over time, and the appearance will improve. The nose will also change in the postoperative period (Fig. 21-5, *B* and *C*). The nose tends to widen and flatten with time. To plan for this, the surgeon will overcorrect the tissues. This will make the nose narrower and higher during surgery.

POSTOPERATIVE CARE

Usually, parents can feed their child after surgery as they did before surgery. Breast-feeding or feeding with nipples will not increase the risk of wound separation.

Parents need to care for the wound meticulously. The lip and nose incisions need to stay clean to prevent wound infection and wound separation. Incisions need to be cleaned frequently and covered by an antibiotic ointment. A team member will show the parents how to do this.

Depending on the surgeon's preference, the sutures in the skin will be removed 5 to 7 days after surgery. Some surgeons prefer to anesthetize the child for suture removal.

Scar Care

Scar care is a long process. Scar stabilization takes more than 6 months. Several methods of scar care are available. Parents will be shown the surgeon's preferred method. Some surgeons prefer to place Micropore tape over the scar to isolate it from the motion of the underlying lip muscle. The parents may be shown how to massage the scar to facilitate scar softening. Additionally, silicone scar sheets can be placed on the scar.

Nasal Splints/Stents

Some surgeons believe that the repaired nose needs help to maintain its shape. Otherwise, the pulling force from the scar will distort the shape. Depending on the technique of surgical repair, a *nasal splint* or nasal stent is useful (Fig. 21-6). It is made of silicone and is available in different sizes. This device may improve the outcome of nasal repair after cleft lip surgery. Similar to the lip scar, the nasal scar takes more than 6 months to stabilize. Depending on the type of surgical repair and the preference of the surgeon, the child may be required to wear the splint for more than 6 months. The splint may be cleaned daily.

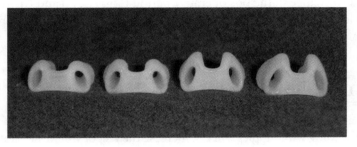

Fig. 21-6   Nasal splints in different sizes.

Most babies adjust to the nasal splint within days. The parents need to tolerate their child's discomfort during this time. During the immediate postoperative period, some children will pull on the lip tape and nasal splint. In an effort to prevent this, the surgeon may require the baby to wear arm restraints to prevent them from hurting the repaired lip and nose.

COMPLICATIONS

All surgical procedures have risks. The possible complications with cleft surgery are the following:

- *Bleeding:* The surgeon will stop all bleeding during surgery, but wound bleeding is possible after surgery. Additional surgery may be required to stop the bleeding.
- *Infection:* Wound infection might result in poor healing, inappropriate scarring, and/or wound separation (very rarely). It is very difficult for the surgeon to reunite the separated parts.
- *Poor scars:* Several factors affect the quality of surgical scars. Wound healing and scar care are factors that affect scar quality. Parents need to care for the wound and scar exactly as instructed by the cleft team. It takes more than 6 months for a scar to mature.
- *Anesthesia:* Although routine anesthesia in otherwise healthy infants and children is very safe, complications can occur and will be discussed by the anesthesiologist.

CONCLUSION

The total rehabilitation of a child with a cleft is a long process. Because the final appearance of the child cannot be determined until facial growth is finished, the surgical outcome will not be truly determined for 17 or 18 years. Fortunately, because of the multidisciplinary approach of team care, children born with clefts receive more efficient and better optimized care than previously available. This translates into fewer surgeries with better outcomes. The most important factor in achieving the best outcome with the fewest surgeries is true collaboration between the patient (when old enough), the family, and the cleft care team.

22

Submucous Cleft Palate

Arun K. Gosain, Steven T. Lanier

KEY POINTS

- A cleft palate results when the two sides of the palate do not fuse together.

- In a cleft palate, a gap is clearly visible in the roof of the mouth.

- A submucous cleft palate is a type of cleft palate that may not be visually apparent, because the muscosa (mouth lining) is intact over the cleft muscles underneath.

- All submucous cleft palates are not the same; they vary in severity.

This chapter focuses on a type of cleft palate, the submucous cleft palate. We discuss how the roof of the mouth, known as the palate, forms during the growth of a fetus. We then describe the characteristics of a submucous cleft palate and the evaluation process used to decide whether a child with a submucous cleft palate requires surgery. Finally, we discuss the various surgeries to correct a submucous cleft palate and what parents can expect after surgery.

BACKGROUND AND HISTORY

The roof of the mouth (palate) forms during the first trimester of pregnancy. The palate initially forms as two halves, known as processes. These processes grow from each side of the mouth, coming together to fuse in the midline. A cleft palate results when these two processes do not grow completely together.

The palate contains two parts, a hard part near the front and a soft part in the back. We make a distinction between these two parts, because they have different functions. The hard palate contains bone covered by mucosa, which is a smooth tissue that lines the entire mouth, and separates the mouth from the nose. The soft palate is made of muscle rather than bone and is very important for swallowing and speech. Children with a cleft palate can have a gap in the bone of the hard palate, atypical formation of the muscles of the soft palate, or both.

In a cleft palate, a gap in the roof of the mouth is clearly visible. In contrast, a submucous cleft palate may not be visually apparent, because the gap in the roof of the mouth is covered by the mucosa that lines the mouth—hence the name "submucous." However, a division of the *uvula,* known as a bifid uvula, may indicate that a submucous cleft palate is present even though it is not visible.

Submucous cleft palates vary in severity. Some children have only a small gap in the hard palate and no differences with the soft palate muscles. Other children have a large gap in the hard palate that is associated with improperly formed soft palate muscles. These children have difficulty with swallowing and speech and need intervention. This difficulty can be an important clue that further testing is needed to evaluate for a submucous cleft palate.

A submucous cleft palate is relatively uncommon, occurring in approximately 1 in 2000 births. The cause is not yet fully understood but probably involves a combination of genetic (inherited) and environmental (exposure of the fetus) factors. Scientists have identified certain genes that are linked to the development of a submucous cleft palate, and a recent study found an increased risk for submucous cleft palate in children of mothers who smoke during pregnancy.

A submucous cleft palate may be the only congenital difference a child has or it may be present in combination with other congenital differences such as a small or large lower jaw, small ears, a cleft lip, and/or fusion of the fingers. When multiple congenital differences are present, genetic testing may be needed to evaluate for the possibility of a genetic syndrome (see Chapter 5). Syndromes associated with submucous cleft palate include velocardiofacial, *Klippel-Feil,* and Treacher Collins.

DIAGNOSIS AND EVALUATION FOR SURGERY

The pediatrician may be able to diagnose a submucous cleft palate by inspecting the baby's mouth. Children with a more subtle form of submucous cleft palate may require more advanced testing for diagnosis. Suspicion for submucous cleft palate is raised when a child has difficulty with swallowing or speech. The term velopharyngeal incompetence (VPI), refers to problems with speech that result from dysfunction of the soft palate muscles (see Chapter 12).

During normal speech, the muscles of the soft palate contract, raising the soft palate and pulling it backward to form a seal against the back of the throat. If this seal does not form because of a problem with the soft palate, food or liquids can enter the nose during feedings. In addition, a child with VPI has a nasal speech quality and difficulty pronouncing certain consonants. To compensate for these difficulties, children with VPI will develop a distinct pattern of pronunciation.

Once VPI is suspected, the single most important test is a formal evaluation by a trained speech-language pathologist (see Chapter 12). Speech-language pathologists use special speech measures and tools to diagnosis VPI. Videofluoroscopy and nasal endoscopy are used to directly visualize the length, height, and motion of the palate. Either method or a combination of the two may be recommended by the team evaluating the child for a submucous cleft palate.

With videofluoroscopy, *radiographs* are taken while the child is swallowing and talking, allowing the examiner to view and measure the movement and shape of the soft palate. With nasal endoscopy, a long, thin, flexible tube with a camera on the end is inserted in the nose, allowing the examiner to directly view the shape and movement of the palate during swallowing and speech. Some centers that treat children with a submucous cleft palate have begun to use magnetic resonance imaging (MRI) to aid in diagnosis and surgical planning. However, more research is needed to determine the usefulness of this method, compared with videofluoroscopy and nasal endoscopy.

TIMING OF SURGERY

Only a small proportion of children with a submucous cleft palate will develop symptoms of VPI. Furthermore, subtle difficulties with speech as a result of a submucous cleft palate may be overcome with speech therapy. Thus, a trial of speech therapy may be beneficial before proceeding with more invasive surgical intervention for VPI. An adequate speech evaluation and a sufficient trial of speech therapy may not be reliably performed before the child is 2½ years of age, and often later. Surgery will be performed as soon as possible after the child is diagnosed with VPI, typically between 2½ and 5 years of age.

OPERATIVE PROCEDURE

The goal of submucous cleft palate surgery is to correct VPI. This is accomplished by lengthening the palate and reconstructing the soft palate muscles. Various surgical techniques can be used. A combination of techniques can be employed, depending on the anatomy of the child's submucous cleft palate. The choice of a particular technique depends on the findings from the clinical evaluation and the surgeon's preference. No one technique is superior in all cases.

Pharyngeal Flap

A pharyngeal flap procedure does not address the submucous cleft palate itself, but rather modifies the back of the throat to improve the seal between the short, dysfunctional palate and the back of the throat during swallowing and speech. It involves raising a piece of muscle and mucosa from the back of the throat and attaching this tissue to the short soft palate. This bridges the large gap between the soft palate and back of the throat. Openings, called lateral ports, are left on either side of the tissue flap to allow continued movement of air from the nose to the throat.

Palatoplasty With Intravelar Veloplasty

Palatoplasty with intravelar veloplasty repositions the malformed soft palate muscles. The most important of these muscles in raising the palate during swallowing and speech is known as the levator veli palatini. This muscle normally raises and moves the palate backward when it contracts. In many submucous cleft palates and in regular cleft palates, the levator veli palatini muscle travels forward to connect to the back of the hard palate, rather than forming a functional, mobile sling by traveling from side to side across the palate. An intravelar veloplasty involves releasing the levator veli palatini from its connection to the hard palate and recreating a muscular sling that travels from side to side across the palate.

Furlow Double-Opposing Z-Plasty

The Furlow double-opposing Z-plasty is a specific kind of palatoplasty that simultaneously lengthens the soft palate while performing an intravelar veloplasty (reorienting the levator speech muscle and reconstructing the speech muscle sling). It involves two Z-shaped incisions in the soft palate that allow a reorientation of the palatal muscles so that they meet at the midline and form a functional sling. The letter Z has a long limb and two short limbs. A cut in the shape of a Z creates two triangular-shaped portions. In a Furlow double-opposing Z-plasty, the long limb of the Z is oriented lengthwise along the soft palate, from front to back. The surgeon cuts along the lines of the Z and rearranges the triangles to reorient the muscle contained in these triangles. The rearrangement not only re-creates the levator sling, but also lengthens the long limb of the Z, thus lengthening the palate.

OUTCOMES AND POTENTIAL COMPLICATIONS

Given that VPI is the primary reason for intervention in patients with a submucous cleft palate, improvement of VPI is the primary outcome measure of the success of an operation. To measure the outcome, the speech-language pathologist repeats a formal speech evaluation after the child has healed and recovered from surgery. The therapist primarily evaluates for improvement in the nasal quality of the child's speech. A high percentage of children with a submucous cleft palate achieve complete resolution of VPI and normalization of speech after surgery. Success rates reported in the literature range from 80% to 97%, and most children do not require further speech therapy.

Complications of surgery to correct a submucous palate can be classified as those that occur shortly after the time of the operation and those that occur later. Possible complications that occur in the short term include bleeding, infection, and wound dehiscence, which involves separation of the wound edges of the repair. In addition, obstructive sleep apnea or hyponasal speech can occur as a result of excessive narrowing of the opening between the nose and the throat, primarily after the pharyngeal flap operation. The rate of these complications is low, and they can be addressed should they occur. However, it is important for families to understand before surgery the risks that are inherent in any surgical procedure and the complications that can occur.

The primary long-term complication of a submucous cleft palate surgery is recurrent VPI. Should patients develop symptoms of recurrent VPI at any point in the postoperative period, then videofluoroscopy and nasal endoscopy are used to assess the movement of the palate and pharyngeal wall and to determine whether the patient might require another operation. An additional, debated potential complication of surgical techniques that involve dissection on the hard palate, such as palatoplasty, is restriction of growth of the maxilla, one of the facial bones that contains the upper teeth. An advantage of techniques that limit surgical dissection of the soft palate, such as the Furlow double-opposing Z-plasty, is that disturbance of the hard palate and potential maxillary growth restriction are avoided.

CONCLUSION

The birth of a new child with a submucous cleft palate can understandably be overwhelming for parents. The evaluation, surgery, and recovery may seem like a long, daunting process. However, parents are not alone in caring for their child. There are many centers with coordinated teams of health care professionals with great experience caring for cleft-affected children. These medical and allied health professionals are dedicated to helping children achieve normal speech and palatal function through modern speech-language therapy and surgical care.

23

Cleft Palate Repair

Gregory D. Pearson, Richard E. Kirschner

KEY POINTS

○ The palate is made of two parts: the hard palate in the front and the soft palate (velum) in the back.

○ A cleft palate leaves an opening between the nose and the mouth that results in feeding and speech difficulties.

○ Palate repair surgery (palatoplasty) helps to correct these problems.

○ Surgical techniques and postoperative management vary depending on the surgeon's preferences.

○ Approximately 10% to 20% of children will need a second surgical procedure to completely correct the function of the palate for speech.

The nose and the mouth are normally separated by the palate, which is made up of the hard palate in the front and the soft palate in the back. The hard palate is composed of *mucous membrane* covering bone, and the soft palate is composed of mucous membrane covering muscle. Before birth, the palate develops as a right half and a left half; these join together at the midline at approximately the third month of pregnancy. When this process does not occur normally, the two sides remain separated, and a cleft palate results. The cleft can involve the soft palate alone or both the soft and hard palate. In other cases, cleft palate can be associated with a cleft of the lip and *alveolus* (gums).

The causes of cleft palate are numerous and cannot always be determined (see Chapter 5). A cleft palate can be linked to inherited causes, including some genetic syndromes, and to maternal risk factors, including the use of some medications (for example, isotretinoin, anticonvulsants, and corticosteroids), smoking, alcohol consumption, diabetes, and folic acid deficiency. In many cases, genetic and environmental factors combine to increase the likelihood of a cleft. Therefore it is usually difficult to name a single factor as the cause of the cleft. A family history of cleft palate, however, is one of the strongest risk factors.

The function of the palate is to separate the mouth from the nose to prevent food and liquid from entering the nasal cavity during swallowing and to prevent the inappropriate escape of air through the nose during speech (hypernasal speech). The soft palate acts as a valve to close off the back of the nose during the production of all speech sounds except "m," "n," and "ng." A properly functioning palate helps speech to be more understandable. To achieve the best speech results, a cleft palate should be repaired before the development of meaningful speech. Therefore, in most centers, palate repair is performed before the child is 12 to 18 months of age.

During normal speech, the soft palate lifts upward and backward to touch the back of the throat (pharynx), thereby closing the valve. A muscle known as the levator veli palatini (levator) normally crosses the interior of the soft palate from side to side, forming a muscular sling that provides the force necessary to lift the soft palate and close the valve. In infants born with a cleft palate, the levator muscle does not form a sling. Instead, the muscle is split, and its two halves run from the front to the back, attaching instead to the back of the cleft hard palate (Fig. 23-1). When surgery is performed, the levator muscle sling is repaired to restore proper functioning of the palate.

Some children may be diagnosed with a submucous cleft palate (SMCP). In children with an SMCP, the palate appears intact but the levator muscles in the soft palate are split. In many children with an SMCP, the uvula is bifid (split in two), a notch can be felt within the back of the hard palate, and a translucent area (zona pellucidum) can be seen in the center of the soft palate. In some children, however, these findings are subtle or absent. Some children with an SMCP require surgical repair. Children with an SMCP can have variable amounts of clefting of the levator muscle. Some have minimal clefting and excellent palatal lift, whereas others have more severe clefting and poor palatal lift. Although typical clefts of the palate need surgical repair in almost all cases, not all submucous clefts require surgery. SMCP is repaired only if it allows inappropriate air escape through the nose during speech (a condition known as velopharyngeal dysfunction, or VPD) because of incomplete closure of the valve. Those with SMCP and normal speech do not require surgical repair. The presence of an asymptomatic SMCP places a child at

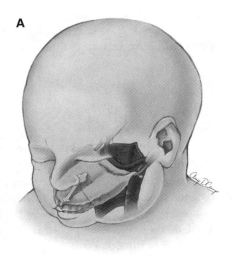

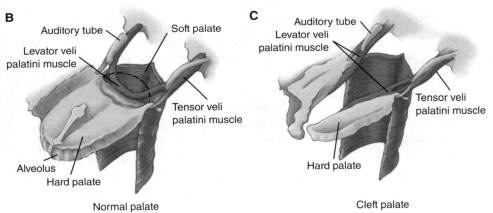

Fig. 23-1 **A** and **B,** Normal anatomy of the palate. **C,** Anatomy of a cleft palate. The levator muscle is incorrectly positioned and attaches to the back edge of the hard palate.

risk for VPD after an adenoidectomy, and this should be considered when an adenoidectomy is recommended. As for all children with clefts, those with SMCP require long-term multidisciplinary team care to properly follow their speech and language development.

Unlike SMCP, overt clefts of the palate (clefts that form an opening between the nose and mouth) require surgical repair in all children except those who are medically unstable or have significant developmental impairment with limited capacity for language development. Surgery for a cleft palate closes the connection between the mouth and nose and repairs the levator muscle sling. Surgical protocols (that is, one- or two-stage repair) and repair techniques may vary from one surgeon to another.

PREOPERATIVE CONSIDERATIONS

Children who have a cleft palate repair require appropriate nutritional intake and weight gain in preparation for the surgery. The infant's weight will be checked frequently before surgery to ensure that nutrition is adequate. Most cleft surgeons perform the palatoplasty when the child is 10 to 12 months of age, although some recommend that surgery be performed slightly earlier or later. For a child with a cleft of the hard and soft palate, the surgeon may perform the palate repair in two stages: the soft palate is repaired in the first stage, and the hard palate is repaired later. Some surgeons believe that delaying repair of the hard palate until the child is older results in improved growth of the upper jaw. This potential advantage, however, must be weighed against the benefit of improved speech results with earlier repair. For this reason, most cleft surgeons prefer to repair the palate in one operation.

Some children with severe developmental delays or other significant medical conditions are better served by postponing or simply not performing palate repair. This decision is made if the risks outweigh the benefits of surgery. Occasionally, a cleft palate repair is delayed because the infant has had a recent cold or respiratory illness. When a child has a significant respiratory illness close to the time of the cleft palate repair, the risk for breathing complications after surgery is increased. Surgery is delayed until after the child has fully recovered from the illness.

SURGICAL PROCEDURES

Several different techniques are available for repairing a cleft palate. All of the tissue needed to complete the repair is present within the palate itself, and no other tissues or materials are added. Dissolving sutures are used so that suture removal is not necessary. Palatoplasty is performed while the child is under general anesthesia and is usually completed in 2 to 3 hours. Most surgeons require patients to stay in the hospital for 1 or 2 days after surgery to ensure that they are feeding well.

The soft palate comprises two layers of mucous membrane, one on the nasal (nose) side and one on the oral (mouth) side of the palate, enveloping the cleft levator muscles. The soft palate can be repaired in either a straight-line or a zigzag manner. The straight-line type of closure is often performed with an *intravelar veloplasty*. In this technique, the muscles are detached from their insertion into the back of the hard palate and sutured to one another to reconstruct the levator muscle sling. The zigzag type of repair is called a *Furlow palatoplasty* (see Fig. 23-2). In this technique, the zigzag closure automatically corrects the position of the levator muscle. This type of repair also lengthens the soft palate. The surgical technique that is used varies according to the cleft type, the surgeon's preference, and institutional protocols.

For clefts of the hard palate, the type of repair varies according to the cleft type and the surgeon's preference. All surgical techniques are designed to repair the mucous membrane on both sides (nasal and oral) of the cleft hard palate. The bone itself is not repaired; closure of the mucous membrane alone is sufficient. To close the mucous membrane, the surgeon must often create relaxing incisions between the palate and gum line to bring the tissues together in the center. This creates openings in the soft tissues just behind the gums that will heal on their own in 2 to 3 weeks. Depending on the surgeon's preference, a two-flap technique may be used, in which the oral tissues are completely released off of the bone and brought together in the midline. Some surgeons use a von Langenbeck technique, in which the tissue is released off the sides but remains attached to the gums in the front of the mouth. Another technique, called the Veau-Wardill-Kilner pushback, completely releases the mucous membrane from the bone, as in the two-flap technique, but also pushes the tissues back toward the soft palate to lengthen the palate. For clefts of the hard palate, mucous membrane from the *nasal septum* (or vomer) may be used to help close the nasal side of the palate.

Fig. 23-2 shows the markings and the steps used in the Furlow technique for repair of a unilateral (one-sided) cleft of the soft and hard palate. Fig. 23-2, *A*, shows the markings for repair of the soft palate and the markings for relaxing incisions to assist with closure of the hard palate. The angled markings on the soft palate will be used to create the zigzag repair and to reconstruct the levator muscle sling. Fig. 23-2, *B*, demonstrates the incisions for lifting the tissue off of the hard palate and the incisions for repairing the soft palate. The improperly oriented levator muscle can be seen within the soft palate. Fig. 23-2, *C*, shows the repair of the nasal mucosa covering the hard palate. Mucous membrane from the nasal septum has been used for closure of the nasal floor. Closure of the triangular flaps of the soft palate reorients the levator muscle into the proper position. Fig. 23-2, *D*, depicts the final

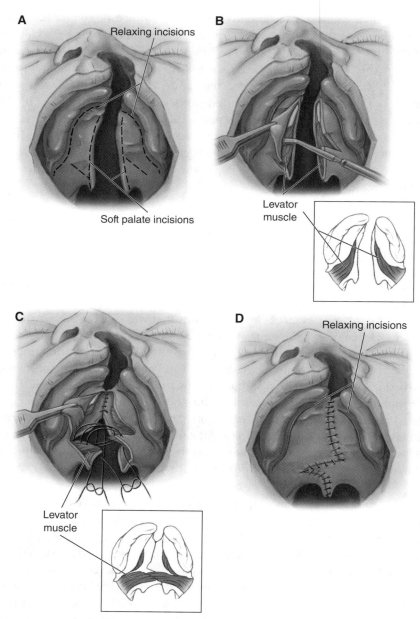

Fig. 23-2   Furlow palatoplasty for repair of a cleft palate. **A,** Markings indicate where incisions will be made. Zigzag incisions will be made within the soft palate, and relaxing incisions will be made on the sides of the hard palate. **B,** The incisions have been made. The incorrectly oriented levator muscle is seen within the soft palate. **C,** The nasal (top) side of the palate is repaired. Repair of the oral (bottom) side of the palate is started. The triangular flaps are sutured to reorient the levator muscle into the proper position. The relaxing incisions are left open. **D,** Final closure of the palate.

closure of the palate. The soft palate is closed in a zigzag pattern, with the levator muscle repaired beneath the mucous membrane. The relaxing incisions in the hard palate are left open and will heal on their own. Closing the cleft in a zigzag fashion lengthens the soft palate.

POSTOPERATIVE CARE

Nearly all infants are admitted to the hospital after surgery. During this time, their breathing, vital signs, and feeding will be closely monitored. Pain medication is given. A small amount of bloody drainage from the mouth and nose is expected, and this usually stops within 24 hours. Feeding protocols (such as the timing, technique, and diet) vary from one institution to another. Some surgeons allow infants to resume using a bottle immediately after surgery. Others prefer that patients use specialty bottles or syringe feedings. Once liquids are tolerated, the diet may be advanced to include soft (stage 2) baby foods. Regardless of the protocol used, most children feed adequately and can be discharged home 1 or 2 days after surgery.

POSTOPERATIVE HOME CARE

After surgery, preventing trauma to the repaired palate is essential. Infants are restricted to a liquid diet and stage 2 baby foods for approximately 3 weeks after surgery. Older children who have undergone palate repair (for example, adopted children and those with SMCP) are restricted to a soft diet until the palate has healed. Children should not use a straw immediately after surgery, because it could damage the palate. Some surgeons allow infants to use a pacifier after surgery, whereas others do not. Finally, many surgeons recommend that infants wear soft arm restraints for 2 to 3 weeks after surgery. These restraints prevent children from placing their fingers and toys in their mouth.

COMPLICATIONS

Children typically have some bloody drainage from their mouth and nose immediately after surgery. Rarely, bleeding is significant, and the child must be returned to the operating room so that the surgeon can find the source of the bleeding and control it. Most children snore immediately after palatoplasty, because the opening between the mouth and nose has now been closed and some swelling is present. Snoring typically resolves within 4 weeks of surgery as the swelling improves. In rare cases, swelling of the palate immediately after surgery may interfere with the child's ability to keep blood oxygen levels normal. These children may require the temporary use of supplemental oxygen and a longer stay in the hospital for monitoring. A very small percentage of children are not able to keep their oxygen levels normal after surgery despite the use of supplemental oxygen. For these children, a breathing tube may be temporarily maintained after surgery. They will be admitted to the intensive care unit for continued monitoring until the tube can be safely removed.

Late complications occur weeks to years after cleft palate repair. If the palate does not heal well, a hole may develop within the line of repair. This connection between the mouth and nose is called an oronasal fistula. A fistula may result from trauma to the repair or from breakdown of the suture line because of excessive tension on the repair. Small palatal fistulas may not cause problems, but larger fistulas can result in leakage of food and fluids from the nose when the child eats and escape of air from the nose when the child speaks. Palatal fistulas will not heal on their own. When they cause problems, surgical repair is needed. The technique and extent of surgery varies depending on the size and location of the fistula.

In some centers, the cleft of the alveolus is repaired at the time of lip repair, a procedure called a *gingivoperiosteoplasty*. In other centers, the cleft within the alveolus is not repaired at the time of the initial lip surgery and is left open until the alveolar bone grafting later in childhood. This results in a temporary connection between the mouth and the nose at the site of the unrepaired alveolus. This type of fistula is not a complication, but rather an intended consequence of the treatment plan. Although this type of fistula may result in some nasal leakage of food or fluids, it usually resolves over time. Fistulas of this type are repaired at the time of alveolar bone grafting.

Even with a properly performed cleft palate repair, 10% to 20 % of children will later demonstrate VPD, usually evident as hypernasal speech. Evaluation of VPD requires the assistance of a specially trained speech-language pathologist and usually requires imaging of the palate during speech (see Chapter 12). VPD will not respond to speech therapy alone. A second operation is necessary to correct the hypernasality and nasal air escape. VPD and oronasal fistulas may or may not have a significant effect on a child's short- or long-term quality of life. When the current or anticipated impact is significant, surgery should be strongly considered.

CONCLUSION

Children with a cleft palate have a connection between the nose and the mouth that results in speech and feeding difficulties. A cleft palate should be repaired by an experienced, specially trained surgeon; the exact method used and postoperative care prescribed vary by surgeon. Approximately 10% to 20% of children will require another procedure after palatoplasty to completely correct their speech.

After the cleft palate repair, the child should be examined regularly by a multidisciplinary cleft team. The team will closely monitor growth and development, speech and hearing, dental health and orthodontic needs, and psychosocial well-being. These regular team visits are the cornerstone of comprehensive cleft care and are essential for achieving the best long-term outcomes.

24

Cleft Lip and Nose Revision

Laura A. Monson, Larry J. Hollier

KEY POINTS

○ Every child with a cleft lip and nose is unique and will have an individualized plan of care.

○ The right surgery and the timing of the surgery are decisions best made by the child, the parents, and the cleft team, together.

○ Some revisions can be performed at almost any time, and others need to be delayed until the child is older or has stopped growing.

○ As children get older, their concerns and wishes should be considered, and they should be involved in the decision-making process.

A cleft lip and palate is associated with specific anatomic differences that affect the lip and nose appearance in predictable ways. The lip and nose are aesthetically prominent facial features, and management of differences in these structures is challenging. Although excellent outcomes can be achieved with the initial procedure, revisions over time are nearly a uniform necessity to maximize facial aesthetics as the child matures and becomes an adult. Patients and their parents can more actively participate in the plan of care if they understand the challenges of cleft surgery and the strategies available to address them.

PREOPERATIVE CONSIDERATIONS

A child born with a cleft lip, with or without a cleft palate, will often need at least one revision or touch-up surgery of the lip and/or nose during his or her lifetime.

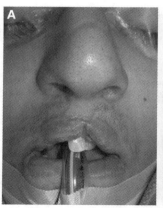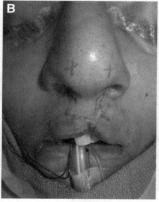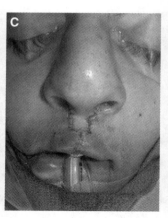

Fig. 24-1 **A,** This child has a significant whistle deformity and is shown before the revision surgery. **B,** The revision is designed. **C,** The child is shown after the revision.

The goal is to produce the most aesthetic appearance possible within the given limits and to restore the child's self-confidence. These efforts should be driven by and in agreement with the child's wishes.

The appearance of a cleft lip and nose can look different from a normal lip and nose. For example, the child with a bilateral cleft lip may have a wide, flat nasal tip; a tight upper lip; and thinness or notching (whistle deformity) of the middle of the red portion (vermilion) of the upper lip. This appearance does not improve with time and can, at least partially, be corrected with surgery (Fig. 24-1).

After the initial cleft lip repair, parents are often concerned about the appearance of the scar. The scar from the first lip repair will take 1 to 1½ years to settle. During this time, thorough scar massage and occasionally special taping will help the appearance of the scar a great deal. It is normal for the scar to be red and thick during the first few months. Sometimes, the scar becomes raised. Problems with the scar may not require a surgery for correction and can often be helped with special tapes or scar massage. Revisions to improve the appearance of the scar should not be considered until at least 1½ years after the original surgery.

One side of the lip may look different from the other side, or asymmetrical. Small differences at the base of the nose or in the red part of the lip can be addressed if they are bothersome to the child, or they can be corrected at a later time. Often, these small touch-ups will be combined with another, larger procedure.

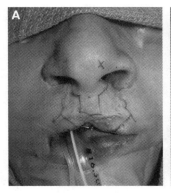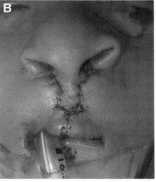

Fig. 24-2   A, This child had a previous cleft repair that resulted in a significant whistle deformity and is shown preoperatively before the revision. **B,** The child is shown postoperatively.

The U-shape of the middle upper lip where the red lip meets the white is called the Cupid's bow. A child born with a cleft does not have this, and the surgeon creates it at the time of the original surgery. The two sides of the Cupid's bow should be level so that they are not noticeable to others at conversational distance. Other small asymmetries of the nose and lip tend to be less obvious. Most cleft surgeons recommend that the Cupid's bow and other asymmetries be revised before the child starts school. Major surgeries such as a formal *rhinoplasty* are often delayed until the child is fully grown, but every effort should be made to make the lip even and the scars as nice as possible before the child enters school. Children start to notice differences between themselves and others and begin teasing when they are approximately 6 years of age (Fig. 24-2).

OPERATIVE PROCEDURES

The upper lip should have an even thickness all the way across or be slightly full in the center. Small notched whistle deformities of the red part of the upper lip can be corrected with minor procedures in which tissue is taken from the lip on either side (Fig. 24-3).

Occasionally, a small amount of fat is taken from the abdomen and used to fill in the area. Larger notches can be more difficult to fix. Sometimes the muscle of the upper lip is not together or is not as tight as it should be, often from stretching over

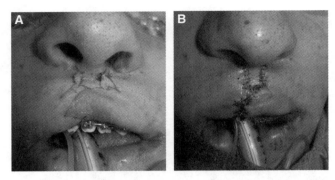

Fig. 24-3   A, This child has asymmetries and is shown before revision surgery. **B,** The patient is shown after surgery.

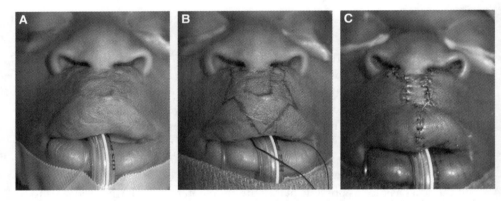

Fig. 24-4   A, This patient has widened scars and is shown before surgery. **B,** The scar revision is designed. **C,** The patient is shown after scar revision and repair of the upper lip muscle, the *orbicularis oris muscle.*

time. For these patients, the surgeon will often recommend that the lip repair be completely redone (Fig. 24-4).

Some patients do not have enough tissue in the rest of the upper lip to transfer. The whole upper lip looks very tight. A lip-switch surgery (Abbé flap) may be needed in which tissue is taken from the lower lip to fill the upper lip (Fig. 24-5). This requires two surgeries and leaves a scar on the lower lip and the chin. This surgery is being performed less often, because our initial care and techniques have improved. Sometimes, however, it is the only way to balance the upper lip and provide enough

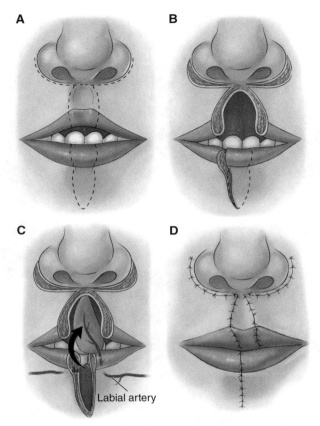

Fig. 24-5 Abbé flap. **A,** Surgical incisions are represented by the dashed lines. **B,** Incisions are made. **C,** The middle part of the lower lip (containing the blood vessel) is transferred to the middle part of the upper lip. **D,** The wounds are closed with stitches and are shown here before they are separated.

tissue. In this procedure, the middle portion of the lower lip is transplanted to the middle part of the upper lip. Its attachment to the lower lip is maintained by one main blood vessel for about 3 weeks, until it begins to receive a new blood supply from the upper lip. Essentially, the middle part of the upper lip is sewn to the middle part of the lower lip. The patient will have a special diet during this time. The attachment between the two lips is then cut or divided.

The area inside the upper lip above the level of the teeth is called the upper *buccal sulcus.* Most people can slide their tongue in front of their teeth and upward into this area. In some children, this area is not deep enough, causing a notice-

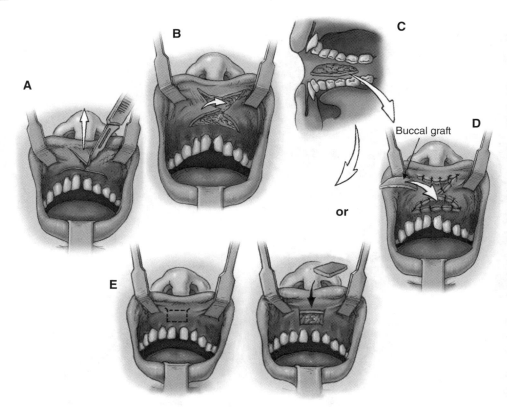

Fig. 24-6   Buccal sulcus release with mucosal graft placement. **A** and **B,** Incisions are made to prepare for transplantation of the graft. **C,** The mucosal graft is taken from another location in the mouth. This area is then sutured closed. **D,** The graft is moved to the new location and sutured in place. **E,** An alternative method is shown.

able difference. The amount of tissue can be insufficient, causing problems with dental appliances and appearance. New tissue needs to be brought into the area to improve its contour. This can be done in two ways. If enough tissue is present on either side, the surgeon can rearrange this tissue to fill the central portion. If there is not enough tissue in the area, a piece of tissue can be grafted from another area. This tissue graft can come from the inside of the cheek as a mucosal graft, or a piece of skin from elsewhere on the body can be taken as a skin graft. This skin will change over time and look more like the inside of the mouth should look, although it will never completely match. When a graft is taken from elsewhere, it has to adhere and take to the new tissue underneath it to receive a blood supply and survive. The surgeon may use special sutures or a molded piece of plasticlike material to keep the graft in place until it is fully healed (Fig. 24-6).

Some children appear to have too much tissue and a bulge that is visible below the lip and over the teeth. These children are often very self-conscious of their smile. In many children, the problem is not that they have too much tissue, but rather the tissue is not attached to the underlying bony gum ridge well. If it is not attached well, it will prolapse or droop when the child smiles. The tissue needs to be resuspended from the bony gum ridge underneath in a much higher position in the buccal sulcus. A plasticlike molded piece of material may be used to keep it in this new position until it heals.

The decision to revise the nose involves more factors than the decision to revise the lip. The nose heals in a less predictable manner than the lip. Every surgery adds more scarring to the nose, which can compromise healing. Most surgeons who perform rhinoplasty find the second rhinoplasty to be much more difficult than the first because of the scarring that resulted from the first surgery. For these reasons, many surgeons recommend delaying rhinoplasty until the child is skeletally mature or has stopped growing. The exception to this general rule is the child who has a severe cleft that causes difficulty breathing or problems with self-esteem and peer interactions. If the problem is small, it is often best to wait until the patient is fully grown so that one definitive surgery is performed, rather than two or more.

Many children with a cleft lip and nose have revision nasal surgery at some time because their nose is asymmetric and the tip lacks projection. The cartilage in the tip of the nose is often insufficient to provide good tip height and definition. The tip of the nose, as well as the base of the nostrils, is often different because the cartilages are splayed and not close enough together in the middle. Many surgeons will use extra cartilage to help build up the nose and provide the needed support. This cartilage can come from the septum of the nose, an ear, or a rib. This can be done in many ways, but the goal is to give strong support to the tip and to correct irregularities and asymmetries. The cartilage that is present may need to be trimmed, excised, or reshaped. Reshaping usually involves placing stitches within the cartilages themselves.

The base of the nose, the distance from the outside of one nostril to outside of the other nostril, is often very wide in a child with a bilateral cleft lip. When the nose is lengthened and has more height, the width improves. However, additional procedures are sometimes required to narrow it further. Tissue can be removed from the inside of the nostril, along the floor of the nose. Sometimes skin can be removed from the outside of the nostril, where the nostril meets the cheek.

The septum of the nose, which separates the nose into two nostrils and nasal passages, is often crooked or deviated. This can lead to obstruction and difficulty breathing. At the time of the rhinoplasty, the septum can be straightened and the misshapen cartilage removed. Sometimes, the cartilage that is removed can be used elsewhere in the nose to help correct other differences.

POSTOPERATIVE CARE AND CONSIDERATIONS

After revision surgery of the lip, patients usually go home the same day. They may need a short course of antibiotic therapy, depending on the surgery that is performed. Care of the stitches and the incision will vary according to the type of stitches placed. Some stitches dissolve and some need to be removed. Two weeks after surgery, scar massage should be started, and special tapes may be prescribed to help with scarring.

After revision surgery of the nose, some patients stay in the hospital overnight. Some are given a short course of oral antibiotic therapy, depending on the type of surgery and whether grafts were used. Care of the incision will depend on the type of stitches that were used. When a lot of work is done on the septum, special plastic stents are placed in the nose to help hold everything in place for the first week after surgery. If the nasal bones are broken and moved at the time of surgery, a plastic splint will be placed on the outside of the nose as well. These will be removed in the clinic the following week. After a major revision surgery of the nose, swelling of the nose and nasal tip can be significant. The surgeon may recommend that the child sleep with the head elevated as much as possible, and sometimes the use of ice packs is advised. The swelling can take many months to completely resolve.

TIMELINE

When is the right time for revision surgery? The preschool years (age 4 to 5 years) are a common time to plan for the first revision of the cleft lip. Asymmetries of the red portion of the lip and widened or thickened scars can be addressed. The lower portion of the nose (nasal tip) can be revised at this time if the difference is significant. Most corrections of the nose are best delayed until the child has stopped growing. At this time, a formal rhinoplasty can be performed. However, the decision about when to have a nose revision is best made together by the parents, the child, and the surgeon. Many children face significant difficulties at school with teasing and bullying because of the appearance of their lip and/or nose. If the nose revision is performed when the patient is a child, the final rhinoplasty will be more difficult and less predictable. However, this might be appropriate for a child who is having problems at school because of bullying. The more precisely children can indicate what bothers them, the greater the likelihood that everyone will be satisfied with the outcome.

COMPLICATIONS

Serious complications are rare after a revision for cleft lip and nose surgery. Infection is probably the most serious complication. Most surgeons prescribe a short course of antibiotic therapy, especially after a major nose revision (involving cartilage grafts). A serious infection that does not respond well to medication by mouth may need to be treated with antibiotics given through an intravenous line or IV. Such an infection is rare. Signs to look for are increasing redness, drainage that smells bad, swelling that is getting worse instead of better, and exquisite tenderness to the touch around the surgical area. The risk of an untreated infection is loss of the cartilage grafts.

Poor scarring can also be considered a complication, although sometimes it cannot be prevented (Fig. 24-7). Some people naturally have a tendency to develop poor scars. After surgery, the scar should continue to improve in appearance and fade in color. Scars that darken in color or become more raised are considered poor scars. Often, the surgeon will prescribe special tapes or possibly injections of steroids to help the scar fade.

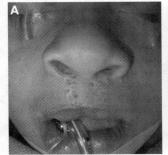
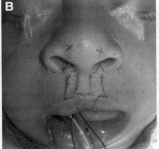
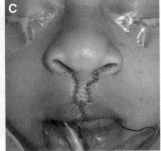

Fig. 24-7   A, This patient has poor scarring and a small whistle deformity and is shown before revision surgery. **B,** The revision is designed. **C,** The child is shown immediately after surgery.

The most common "complication" after a revision of a cleft lip and nose is probably a result that is not desired. Sometimes the appearance is not what the patient and family had hoped for. These surgeries are challenging. Parents need to have an open and frank discussion about this with the surgeon before surgery. As mentioned previously, the likelihood of satisfaction with the surgical outcome is increased when the child can specifically indicate the things that are bothersome.

CONCLUSION

Cleft lip and nose repair is a powerful surgery that is very effective in improving the appearance of a child with a cleft. These procedures, however, are technically demanding and their results are not perfect; revision surgery is frequently required over time. The sequence and timing of revision procedures are based on the concerns of the patient and family and the child's psychosocial situation and level of skeletal maturity. When these factors are thoroughly considered and all parties have reasonable expectations, excellent outcomes often are achieved.

25

Surgery for Velopharyngeal Dysfunction

Paula G. Klaiman, Simone J. Fischbach, Christopher R. Forrest

---

KEY POINTS

○ In some children with a cleft palate, too much air escapes through the nose during speech, causing velopharyngeal dysfunction (VPD) and hypernasality.

○ VPD can occur for several reasons in patients with a cleft; proper treatment depends on an accurate diagnosis.

○ Treatment for VPD consists of speech therapy and/or surgery, which modifies the palate or the throat to improve the velopharyngeal valve.

○ Approximately 20% of children who have palatoplasty will require surgery to correct VPD later in childhood, despite an excellent surgical technique.

This chapter explains why cleft-affected children need surgery to correct nasal-sounding speech (hypernasality) and describes the different surgical options. Hypernasality occurs when too much sound and air pass through the nose during speech. In English, sounds and air pass only through the mouth, except for the sounds m, n, and ng, which move through the nose. All other sounds in English are oral sounds and are produced by sound and air directed through the mouth.

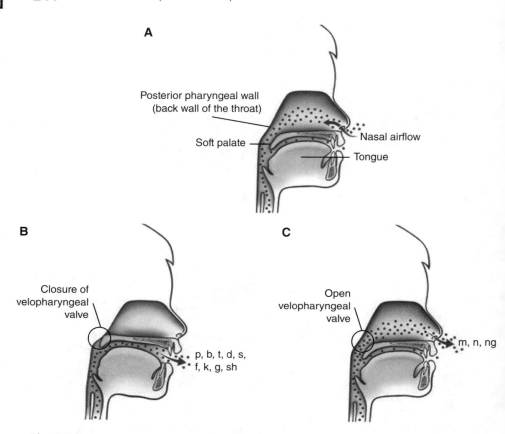

Fig. 25-1   A, During rest and breathing, the velopharyngeal valve (created by the velum or soft palate and the posterior pharyngeal wall [back of the throat]) is open, allowing for nasal airflow. **B,** When making oral sounds, the velopharyngeal valve is closed to prevent nasal air escape. **C,** When making nasal sounds, the velopharyngeal valve is open to allow nasal air escape.

This is possible because the soft palate (velum) rises up and contacts the back wall of the throat (posterior pharyngeal wall) while the side walls of the throat (lateral pharyngeal walls) come together. This creates a velopharyngeal valve to close off the nose from the mouth during speech and swallowing (Fig. 25-1). When velopharyngeal closure does not occur correctly during speech, it is referred to as velopharyngeal dysfunction (VPD) and results in hypernasality. VPD is also known as velopharyngeal insufficiency, velopharyngeal inadequacy, and velopharyngeal incompetency (VPI).

VPD occurs for several reasons. In a child with a repaired cleft palate, the soft palate may be too short to contact the back of the throat and/or the muscles of the soft palate do not function properly. Despite the best possible care, most centers report approximately a 20% likelihood that a child born with a cleft palate will need another secondary surgery to correct hypernasality after the repair of the cleft palate.

To minimize the need for surgery to treat VPD, the child's cleft palate should be repaired early. Most centers surgically repair a cleft palate in children 9 to 12 months of age unless medical reasons necessitate delaying surgery. Care by a team of specialists who have experience with cleft-affected children is essential. The speech-language pathologist will provide suggestions and activities to engage the child in early development of speech sounds and the use of more words. The therapist will also help parents to recognize when their child is making unusual speech sounds (compensatory misarticulations) and how to react to discourage their continued use. These efforts assist in determining whether the child's speech is hypernasal and when more detailed testing is needed.

TIMELINE

By 3 to 4 years of age, children talk in short sentences and are usually cooperative enough to provide a speech sample that can be evaluated for hypernasality. The speech-language pathologist will listen to the child's speech and determine the potential for producing better speech with therapy or whether the child should be referred for further testing to assess the muscles of the soft palate.

The muscles and structures of the velopharyngeal valve can be tested by nasopharyngoscopy and/or *multiview videofluoroscopy*. Briefly, nasopharyngoscopy involves inserting a small fiberoptic tube (endoscope) into one nostril to view the soft palate and surrounding structures from above. Multiview videofluoroscopy is an X-ray test in which the inside of the nose is coated with barium (white chalky liquid). This helps the examiner see the structures more clearly on video X-ray pictures while the child talks. For either of these tests, the child is asked to repeat selected sounds, words, and sentences. The examiner can determine whether the velopharyngeal valve closes correctly during oral speech or whether a gap or opening causes sound and air to leak into the nose, or VPD. When surgery is recommended, the information from these tests guides the surgeon in choosing the procedure that will provide the best possible result.

PREOPERATIVE CONSIDERATIONS

Several factors need to be considered to determine whether the child requires surgery and to select the best procedure. Input from several specialists may be needed.

Medical History

The surgeon will review the child's medical history to determine whether further testing is needed before the surgery is performed. This includes information about airway obstruction (tonsils, adenoids, and sleep apnea and/or difficulty breathing when sleeping), past surgeries, and other medical conditions that might be relevant. In addition, an anesthesia consultation may be recommended for children with more complex medical histories. Some patients are not good candidates for VPD surgery. For these children, a prosthetic appliance may be recommended to help improve the functioning of the soft palate.

The presence, size, and location of the gap in the velopharyngeal valve, as well as the pattern of muscle movement in the pharynx, are determined by analyzing information from nasopharyngoscopy and/or multiview videofluoroscopy. This information is used to determine whether to lengthen or rerepair the soft palate (Furlow palatoplasty) or narrow the gap with a pharyngoplasty (pharyngeal flap pharyngoplasty or sphincter pharyngoplasty), both of which are described later in the chapter.

Surgeon's Experience and Preference

Each center has a preferred type of surgery based on the surgeons' experience and expertise. Current research on the success of VPD procedures shows that when the surgeon is experienced in cleft palate surgery, no single procedure is favored. However, the best choice is the least invasive and least risky procedure that will most likely result in the best possible speech outcomes.

Parental and Patient Concerns

Parents have to make a very personal decision when considering surgery to correct their child's nasal speech. Some children are very aware that their speech is different and are teased by others, and some children become frustrated. Other children lack this awareness of their speech difference, but people around them make comments about it. VPD can also lead to other speech differences such as difficulty producing speech sounds (compensatory misarticulation) and voice problems such as a soft and/or hoarse voice. The child might not be understood by others because of these difficulties. Surgery is recommended only when normal-sounding speech is not possible with speech therapy alone.

OPERATIVE PROCEDURES

Two options are available for surgical correction of VPD:
- Lengthening or rerepair of the soft palate (Furlow palatoplasty or Z-plasty)
- Narrowing of the velopharyngeal gap (pharyngeal flap pharyngoplasty, sphincter pharyngoplasty, and pharyngeal wall augmentation)

All of these procedures are performed inside the mouth while the child is asleep under general anesthesia. After surgery, the child will be taken to the recovery room and closely monitored before being moved onto the ward. The surgeon will provide parents with information about the length of the operation and the duration of their child's stay in the hospital.

Lengthening Procedures

Lengthening procedures or rerepair of the soft palate can be successful in managing VPD in certain circumstances. These procedures are typically selected when the size of the velopharyngeal gap is small. A common lengthening procedure is the Furlow palatoplasty or Z-plasty (Fig. 25-2). It leaves a Z-shaped scar on the soft palate. A Z-shaped incision is made on both the oral and nasal side of the soft palate, and the tissue/muscles are rotated. The tissues are moved so that the orientation of the velopharyngeal muscles is more appropriate. This rearrangement improves the movement of and lengthens the soft palate, helping it to contact the back wall of the throat and prevent air and sound from escaping through the nose

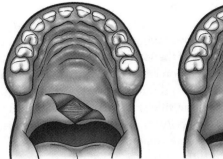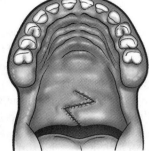

Fig. 25-2   Furlow palatoplasty.

inappropriately. The advantage of this operation is a decreased risk of developing nasal airway obstruction and breathing difficulties when sleeping (obstructive sleep apnea). This procedure can also be used as an initial surgical approach for treating VPD in selected children; if results are not optimal after monitoring and additional therapy, the child can have a different surgery (pharyngeal flap pharyngoplasty or sphincter pharyngoplasty) to further correct the problem.

Potential Complications

A possible but rare complication of Furlow palatoplasty or Z-plasty is a breakdown along the suture lines, which can result in a small hole (palatal fistula). This may require another surgery to repair the hole if it affects speech or if liquid escapes through the nose when the child drinks. As with any surgery inside the mouth, bleeding and infection can occur. These occurrences are rare and can be treated.

Narrowing the Velopharyngeal Gap

Another group of operations is designed to correct VPD by adding tissue to narrow the gap between the soft palate and the back of the throat. Tissue is taken either from the back of the throat (pharyngeal flap pharyngoplasty) or from the side walls of the throat (sphincter pharyngoplasty).

A method that is rarely used in children is augmentation of the posterior pharyngeal wall with implants or injectable materials. Augmentation procedures have several disadvantages. Injectable materials can be absorbed, they often move from the location where they were initially placed, and they can become infected. The procedure may need to be repeated several times to obtain the desired results, making this a poor option for children.

The pharyngeal flap procedure involves taking a strip of tissue from the back of the throat and attaching it to the center of the soft palate (Fig. 25-3). After surgery, two small holes (lateral ports) are present on either side, which allow nasal breathing, drainage of nasal mucus, and correct production of nasal sounds (m, n, and ng). When oral sounds are produced, the side walls (lateral pharyngeal walls) move against the flap to close both lateral ports, thereby eliminating hypernasality. The width of the flap is determined by analyzing information from visualization techniques (nasopharyngoscopy and/or multiview videofluoroscopy). The success of the procedure depends not only on ensuring that the width and location of the flap are appropriate, but also on the ability of the lateral walls to move against it. The earlier the pharyngeal flap surgery is performed, the faster the child's speech will improve.

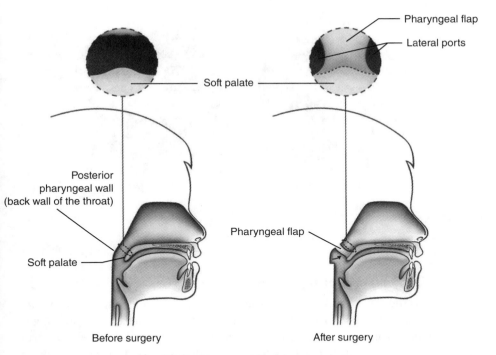

Fig. 25-3   Pharyngeal flap pharyngoplasty.

A sphincter pharyngoplasty changes the shape of the velopharyngeal space, but in a different way compared with pharyngeal flap pharyngoplasty (Fig. 25-4). The sphincter procedure is designed to create a muscular circle (sphincter) that leaves a smaller velopharyngeal opening in the center of the throat. This procedure is recommended and tends to work best when movement of the sides of the throat (lateral pharyngeal walls) is poor. In this procedure, tissue is raised with muscle from both sides of the throat and inserted into the back wall of the throat (posterior pharyngeal wall). This is done at the level where the soft palate attempts to contact the posterior pharyngeal wall. Some surgeons recommend removal of the tonsils and adenoids a few months before surgery to allow better positioning and insertion of the flaps. A sphincter pharyngoplasty is usually performed on both sides (bilateral), but it can be done on one side (unilateral). The sphincter creates one hole in the middle surrounded by flaps of tissue, whereas the pharyngeal flap creates two holes, one on each side of the throat.

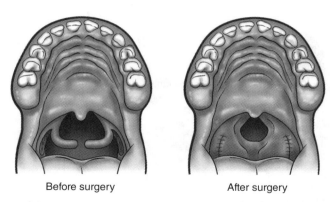

Before surgery   After surgery

Fig. 25-4   Sphincter pharyngoplasty.

Potential Complications

Snoring is the most common undesirable consequence of pharyngoplasty surgeries. This is most obvious immediately after surgery when expected swelling is
present, but it can continue to some extent for the rest of the child's life. In a small
number of patients, the flap may be too wide or the sphincter too small, resulting
in obstructive sleep apnea. Signs of this difficulty include a combination of severe
snoring, pauses or absence of breathing during sleep, bed-wetting, excessive daytime sleepiness/sluggishness, and changes in personality or behavior (irritability,
hyperactivity, depression, poor concentration, and learning problems). Signs of
obstructive sleep apnea are common in the immediate postoperative period but
should be reported to the surgeon if they persist. In some cases, the surgeon may
decide to return the child to the operating room to revise the pharyngoplasty.
Rarely, a pharyngeal flap or sphincter needs to be taken down or removed. The
child may have difficulty clearing nasal mucus, particularly when he or she has a
cold. This can be managed with nasal decongestants and/or saline sprays.

Another possible side effect is overcorrection or undercorrection of VPD. Overcorrection can occur if the flap is too wide or the sphincter is too small, causing
the child to sound like he or she has a cold *(hyponasal).* Undercorrection results if
the pharyngeal flap is too narrow or the hole created in sphincter pharyngoplasty
does not close properly during speech. Pharyngeal and sphincter flaps that are
placed too low can result in a degree of continued hypernasality. The cleft palate
team will determine whether further revision surgery is necessary.

In rare cases, infection, bleeding, and wound-healing problems (fistula or flap breakdown) can be a problem after pharyngoplasty surgery.

POSTOPERATIVE CARE AND CONSIDERATIONS

Children occasionally have throat and/or neck pain after surgery. This results from surgery to the soft palate and positioning of the neck during the operation. The child cannot take medicine by mouth immediately after the surgery. Pain medicine is given through an intravenous line to keep the child comfortable. The pain generally subsides after a few days.

The child cannot eat or drink immediately after surgery. Intravenous fluids usually are given until the child can drink an adequate amount of liquids. Once the child is drinking well and is comfortable taking oral pain medication, he or she will be discharged from the hospital. The stitches in the palate and throat usually dissolve a few weeks after surgery. A soft diet is required for several weeks after the operation until the incision lines are completely healed. Parents are given a list of foods and liquids that their child can and cannot have. Eating and drinking are essential to speed healing.

The incision needs to remain clean. The child's mouth should be rinsed with water after all feedings and drinking, including after taking liquid medicine. Parents can assist with brushing their child's teeth gently a few days after surgery, making sure that the toothbrush is not too far back in the throat, near the incisions.

The corners of the child's mouth may be red or sore, because the mouth has been stretched during surgery. This will heal quickly, and Vaseline can be applied to the corners of the mouth to help reduce soreness. Physical activity should be limited during the first few weeks after surgery to prevent accidental injury to the mouth and to promote healing.

Parents should call the child's doctor immediately if their child:
- Is not eating or drinking
- Has a fever
- Is bleeding from the mouth
- Has a foul odor from the mouth
- Is gasping for air when sleeping and waking frequently throughout the night (obstructive sleep apnea)

In many patients, reduction in the nasal quality of the voice is noticed shortly after surgery. However, children who continue to have incorrect speech patterns (compensatory articulations) may require more time and speech therapy. The speech-language pathologist will teach the child how to make sounds correctly and how to control nasal speech after surgery. This requires a commitment from the therapist, the child, and the parents. Consistent and frequent practice results in faster and better improvement.

Parents should follow all postoperative care instructions provided by the center and attend all scheduled follow-up visits with their child so that the speech-language pathologist and surgeon can assess the outcome of the surgery, continue to make recommendations for care, and address all questions and concerns.

Part VI

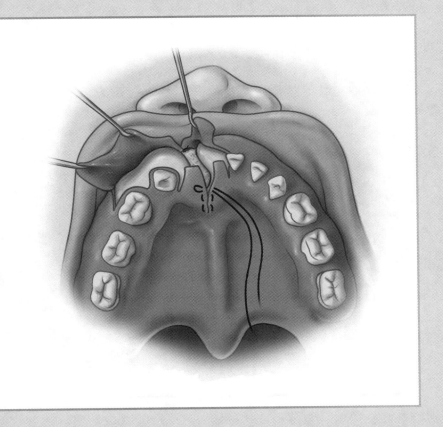

Cleft Palate Dental
and Orthodontic Principles

26

Pediatric Dentistry

Donald V. Huebener

KEY POINTS

- The pediatric dentist has a unique role on the cleft team, providing checkups, preventive care, placement of fillings, and orthodontic care.

- The first dental visit for a child with a cleft is usually just after birth.

- Pediatric dental care is usually provided in four stages:
  - Stage I: Initial management (birth to 2½ years of age)
  - Stage II: Primary *dentition* (2½ to 6 years of age)
  - Stage III: Mixed dentition (6 to 12 years of age)
  - Stage IV Permanent dentition (12 years of age to the late teen years)

$C$are for an infant with a cleft is best provided by a group of doctors and other specialists who work together on a cleft team (see Chapter 1). The cleft team consists of four dental specialists who perform diagnostic and direct care of patients: (1) the pediatric dentist provides routine oral health care, (2) the orthodontist provides braces, (3) the prosthodontist performs tooth replacements, and (4) the oral surgeon performs tooth extractions and sometimes assists with alveolar bone grafting (see Chapter 29) and jaw surgery. Each specialist follows the guidelines set forth by the American Cleft Palate-Craniofacial Association and works closely with the other medical and allied specialists, such as the speech-language therapist and the audiologist, to provide the best and most current multidisciplinary care.

Pediatric dentists are unique members of the team. They provide routine oral health care (checkups, placement of fillings, orthodontic care, and preventive services) from birth through late adolescence. The American Academy of Pediatric Dentistry suggests that infants be seen for their first visit after the first baby tooth comes in or before 1 year of age. For infants with a cleft, the first dental visit should occur usually right after birth to provide optimal dental care. Early care includes preventive and restorative dental care to meet the needs of cleft-affected children. These needs are similar to those of children without a cleft. However, care for children with a cleft also focuses on special procedures and collaboration with other team members for cleft lip/palate management.

SEQUENCING: GETTING STARTED AND WHAT'S NEXT

In general, the timing of dental interventions for infants with clefts is related to the development of the *primary teeth* and the *permanent teeth,* along with the growth of the head and face. These interventions proceed in an orderly fashion with treatments from other health care providers and are part of the overall team protocol. Dental procedures are performed during four classical stages related to the patient's age and dental development. Stage I is the initial management stage, stage II is the primary dentition stage, stage III is the mixed dentition stage, and stage IV is the permanent dentition stage. The medical specialist and other specialists perform procedures during these stages according to the team recommendations.

Stage I: Initial Management

Stage I spans the time from birth to 2½ years of age. Shortly after birth, the pediatric dentist, the plastic surgeon, and the nurse feeding specialist see the newborn infant with a cleft. At the first visit, the child may be seen by other team members or by a few specialists. The infant's nutrition and the first surgical procedure to restore the nose and lip are discussed. The nurse feeding specialist instructs the parents on the methods of feeding their infant. Most newborns receive adequate nutrition with assisted feeding. For some children, the pediatric dentist will make an acrylic feeding appliance to help with feeding. The appliance is constructed on plaster models of the infant's mouth. It is placed on the roof of the mouth and allows food and liquids to enter the digestive tract properly and safely.

During stage I, the use of a presurgical cleft appliance is discussed with the parents (see Chapter 27). Various intraoral (inside the mouth) and extraoral (outside the mouth) appliances have been developed to help correct the cleft and assist the surgeon before the initial lip surgery. Presurgical appliances can help the surgeon obtain a better cleft repair and improve the surgical outcome. An example of this type of appliance is the nasoalveolar molding (NAM) appliance, which assists in improving the contour of the nose and the upper jaw before surgery. The cleft team will use other types of appliances before and after surgery, depending on the team philosophy and protocols they have developed. Many teams do not use any type of infant appliances and obtain excellent results.

If a NAM appliance is planned, the pediatric dentist (or sometimes the orthodontist) will obtain a dental impression (model) of the cleft upper jaw and make a plaster cast to construct the appliance. In the second visit with the pediatric dentist, the NAM appliance is placed, and parents are given instructions for its use. Subsequent appointments are made. During the next appointments, the appliance is adjusted and any necessary modifications performed. When the desired outcome is achieved, the pediatric dentist will inform the plastic surgeon that the infant is ready for the initial lip closure.

The pediatric dentist begins the infant oral health care program in stage I. This program, advocated by the American Academy of Pediatric Dentistry, is designed to provide guidance to parents regarding the eruption of the primary teeth, the prevention of dental *caries,* the initiation of toothbrushing and techniques, flossing, the use of fluorides, and injuries to the teeth. In addition, for infants with a cleft, the dental conditions associated with cleft lip/palate are discussed with the parents. These concerns include congenitally missing teeth (teeth not present at birth), teeth in the cleft area, *supernumerary teeth,* malformed teeth, and teeth that are not in the normal position. Other concerns are discussed, including the timing of orthodontics, bone grafting, the replacement of congenitally missing teeth, and the need for routine dental checkups by the pediatric dentist, from the child's infancy to the late teen years. Finally, the pediatric dentist reviews the important aspects of good oral hygiene and prevention of dental caries in the primary teeth. Healthy primary teeth are needed for good speech, aesthetics, chewing, and the proper eruption of the permanent teeth.

Stage II: Primary Dentition

Stage II occurs when the child is 2½ to 6 years of age. The primary teeth usually begin to erupt at 6 to 8 months of age in the following order:
- Lower central incisors
- Upper central incisors 1 month later
- Lateral incisors
- Primary first molars
- Primary second molars

By the time the child is 2½ years of age, all primary teeth should be present. Many parents note that during the eruption process (teething), their child has increased salivation (drooling) and places his or her hand in the mouth frequently. Teething can cause daytime restlessness and some loss of appetite. Research has shown that teething does not cause a fever, diarrhea, convulsions, sleep disturbance, infections, croup, or other illnesses. It is a normal process and may cause slight soreness around erupting teeth as they emerge through the gums. This soreness usually subsides within a few days. Parents and other caregivers need to be aware of the following information about rubbing an anesthetic medicine (medicine that numbs or causes a decreased sensation) over the gums as teeth emerge. On June 26, 2014, the Food and Drug Administration (FDA) warned caregivers not to prescribe topical viscous lidocaine for symptoms relating to tooth eruption. In addition, the FDA warned parents and caregivers not to use over-the-counter topical medications for teething pain because some of them can be harmful. Parents should discuss these products with their child's doctor and/or members of the cleft team if they have questions or concerns.

The primary dentition stage extends from 2½ years of age, when all of the primary teeth should have erupted into the mouth, until about 6 years of age, when the permanent mandibular incisors in the lower arch come in. This is the beginning of the mixed dentition stage, which is characterized by the presence of both primary and permanent teeth. Cleft-affected children often have a delay in eruption of teeth on the cleft side. Some children with a cleft may never form certain teeth, especially in the lateral incisor area. *Enamel* and/or *dentin* defects can be present on teeth close to the actual cleft area. Extra primary teeth can be present in the cleft area, and some of these teeth can erupt into the cleft or along the side of the cleft. Usually, removal of these teeth is delayed unless they have tooth decay that is too severe for repair or they interfere with permanent tooth development.

After all of the primary teeth erupt, the child's occlusion (bite) can be examined. This is the manner in which the maxillary teeth (teeth in the upper jaw) and the mandibular teeth (teeth in the lower jaw) come together. In cleft children, the occlusion may be different. A left-right mismatch between the upper and lower tooth positions or an overbite or underbite can occur. A *crossbite* can be present in the anterior area (front of the mouth) or in the posterior area (back of the mouth); they can be unilateral (present on one side of the mouth) or bilateral (present on both sides of the mouth). Primary teeth can be rotated, tipped, and malpositioned, especially on the cleft side. The correction of misaligned primary teeth is based on the cleft team's philosophy, treatment protocols, and the child's cooperation. Usually, the teeth are moved when the permanent teeth begin to erupt. An orthodontist places braces or other appliances to do this. In some children, however, the misaligned teeth may need to be moved earlier to the correct position.

During the primary dentition stage, children should begin to have routine dental care at 6-month intervals (dental checkups) with the pediatric dentist. These periodic dental visits are necessary to help ensure the health of the primary teeth and the oral health in general. Primary teeth are important for chewing, aesthetics, and speech. They assist in guiding the permanent teeth into their proper place in the dental arches. During the dental checkup, the oral cavity is examined and different conditions are noted. If caries are present, a restorative treatment plan is established. Good oral hygiene practices and preventive measures that can be performed at home are discussed. A thorough cleaning and fluoride treatment are performed. Finally, the parents' questions are answered, and all concerns are discussed.

Stage III: Mixed Dentition

The mixed dentition stage occurs when the child is 6 to 12 years of age. It begins with the eruption of the mandibular permanent incisors and continues until the permanent maxillary canines appear—the last permanent teeth to erupt, with the exception of the third molars (wisdom teeth). During this time, primary and permanent teeth are present in the mouth at the same time. With the permanent teeth present, orthodontic correction can begin.

Several medical and dental interventions begin in stage III, including phase I orthodontic correction (correction of crossbite and anterior maxillary incisor alignment), secondary alveolar bone grafting, and temporary replacement of missing permanent teeth in the front of the upper jaw. In general, phase I orthodontic correction precedes the surgical alveolar bone grafting procedure. Frequently, maxillary incisors in the area next to the cleft erupt rotated and out of alignment. These anterior teeth are moved into a more desirable position to allow successful bone grafting. At the same time, the *posterior crossbite* is corrected. Timing of the first phase of orthodontic correction depends on the eruption of the permanent first molars (necessary for placement of orthodontic brackets/bands for the appliance) and the maxillary incisors (also necessary for the placement of brackets). Usually, the first phase of orthodontics can begin when the child is 8 to 8½ years of age and is completed within approximately 1 year depending on the child's cooperation. Parents and caregivers will notice a welcomed change in facial appearance and tooth position at this time. If the lateral incisor (in a unilateral cleft) or both lateral incisors (in a bilateral cleft) are congenitally missing, space will be made for a *pontic* to allow a normal number of anterior maxillary teeth when braces are completed. Sometimes the orthodontist will recommend closure of the space where a permanent tooth is missing. This decision depends on the relationship of the *maxilla* to the mandible and the presence or absence of other permanent teeth and their position.

Once the first phase of braces is complete, the orthodontist will notify the plastic surgeon or *oral surgeon* that the teeth are in proper position for the next procedure, the alveolar bone graft. Bone grafting in both unilateral and bilateral complete cleft lip and palate patients is necessary to strengthen the part of the upper jaw that supports the teeth (alveolus) and to allow the lateral incisor (if present) and the canine to erupt through bone. These processes improve periodontal health. In addition, bone grafting helps to support future dental implants that will be needed if a tooth or teeth never develop. Finally, the grafting procedure contours the alveolus, providing a more normal shape for pontic placement.

After the alveolar bone graft is completed, the patient with a cleft sees the orthodontist, who will place an orthodontic retainer to maintain the new position of the teeth while the bone graft matures. If any teeth do not develop, the orthodontist will place pontics on the retainer as replacements for teeth in the front of the upper jaw. The patient wears the retainer until the second phase of full-banded orthodontic braces can begin, after eruption of the rest of the permanent teeth (with the exception of the wisdom teeth).

Oral health care and routine dental checkups are very important in stage III. The risk of developing caries and gingival (gum) inflammation increases with the placement of orthodontic appliances. Plaque and bacteria, which contribute to the development of caries, live and grow near orthodontic bands, brackets, and arch wires. Both the orthodontist and the pediatric dentist stress the importance of good toothbrushing and effective home care instructions. Additionally, in the cleft area, rotated teeth and the irregular shape of the cleft alveolus harbor bacteria and plaque, making toothbrushing and oral hygiene even more important. Effective toothbrushing techniques along with appropriate topical fluoride therapy will help to minimize the possibility of tooth decay. Dental sealants placed on the occlusal (biting) surfaces of 6- and 12-year molars may help to further reduce the risk for dental caries. Consuming fewer sugary foods and drinks contributes to reducing tooth decay.

Stage IV: Permanent Dentition

Stage IV occurs when the child is 13 to 18 years of age. This stage begins with the full eruption of the premolars and canines; all teeth are present at this point except the wisdom teeth. The orthodontist reevaluates the growth of the maxilla and mandible and the way in which the upper jaw and lower jaw come together. In most patients, cleft orthodontic conditions can be corrected with conventional braces. The treatment period is approximately 21 to 24 months, depending on the child's cooperation. After active orthodontic treatment, retainers are placed to help manage empty spaces created by missing teeth until a permanent replacement tooth is placed.

Some patients with clefts will require a more extensive treatment approach to place the maxilla and mandible into the proper position and occlusion. Genetics and environmental factors both contribute to the amount of growth achieved by the maxilla. In some children, maxillary growth may be so reduced that it is too far behind the mandible to be corrected by orthodontic treatment alone. In these cases, a surgical-orthodontic approach is necessary to realign the dental arches. Close cooperation by team members is critical to the success of a combined approach. First, the orthodontist aligns the teeth in both arches and straightens the dentition. Next, the plastic or oral surgeon repositions to the upper and lower jaw to improve the relationship between them. These surgical procedures are performed after facial growth is complete. Usually, this will occur in females at approximately 15 to 16 years of age and in males after 18 years of age. After surgery and with the braces still in place, the orthodontist will make final adjustments to the teeth and the dental arches. When the desired outcome is achieved, the orthodontist will remove the appliances and construct retainers (with pontics to replace missing teeth, if necessary) to hold the teeth and dental arches in their new position.

Good oral health care is critical during both phases of orthodontic treatment. Much information is available about oral hygiene, plaque, and dental caries during the course of orthodontic therapy. Orthodontic brackets, bands, wires, and other tooth-movement hardware are ideal places for microorganisms that can cause cavities. Sugar-containing foods and drinks increase the risk of tooth decay. Effective toothbrushing techniques coupled with good dietary habits will help to decrease the risk of tooth decay. Supplemental topical fluoride therapy is also important.

The pediatric dentist and the orthodontist communicate closely and on a regular basis during stage IV. A complete periodic oral examination with appropriate dental X-ray images, a thorough cleaning, and a fluoride treatment should be performed before the placement of orthodontic appliances. In addition, if sealants on permanent molars are to be used, they should be placed before braces are placed. While the child wears braces, continued checkups are needed every 6 months (and more frequently, if necessary). Cleanings and fluoride treatments are performed at these appointments. Toothbrushing should be performed at least twice a day with a fluoride-containing toothpaste. This helps to remove plaques and microorganisms from around the orthodontic appliances and decreases the risk of tooth decay. Brushing three times a day is preferred. If cavities develop during active orthodontic therapy, they should be treated immediately and oral hygiene and toothbrushing reinforced.

Finally, after orthodontic therapy is complete and retainers are in place, missing teeth can be addressed. Retainers are placed, with pontics in position for all missing teeth. This is a temporary measure designed for better aesthetics and space management until the late teen years or early adulthood, when a decision about permanent replacement is made. In general, *prosthodontists* and adult general dentists perform these replacements. Several options are available:

- Fixed prosthodontic: A bridge with a pontic placed in the cleft area
- Maryland bridge: A bridge that minimally involves the preparation of adjacent teeth in the cleft area
- Implant: A device placed in the cleft area bone on which a pontic is placed
- Acrylic palatal retainer: A removable device with a pontic placed in the position of the missing tooth

Each method of tooth replacement has advantages and disadvantages, and many factors should be considered. For example, "Is there enough bone in the cleft site to support an implant?" This and other questions are discussed between the patient, the parents, and the practitioner who will perform the procedure.

CONCLUSION

Pediatric dentists on cleft teams help to ensure that patients with clefts receive the appropriate dental care. They continue to provide care until patients are in their late teens to ensure the most desirable outcome. Dental care for infants with clefts should begin shortly after birth and continue until the late teen years. Routine dental care is important to maintain optimal oral health in all stages of cleft care. The sequencing of treatment proceeds in an orderly manner and in part is related to the patient's age and dental development. The pediatric dentist, in coordination with other team members, performs specific treatment protocols in correcting the patient's cleft.

27

Presurgical Infant Orthopedics and Nasoalveolar Molding

Osama A. Basri, Lindsay A. Schuster

KEY POINTS

- Some cleft treatment centers perform a technique called presurgical infant orthopedics (PSIO) during the first months of the infant's life to reduce the severity of clefting in preparation for the child's first lip and nose surgery.

- The aim of PSIO is to narrow the cleft, reducing the gap in the alveolar segments (gum pads) and lips. Some techniques also treat the anatomy of the cleft-affected nose.

- Multiple PSIO techniques exist, including lip taping, the Latham appliance, and nasoalveolar molding (NAM). Lip adhesion is a surgical alternative that temporarily closes the cleft in the lip and molds the gum pads together before the definitive lip and nose surgery.

- Typically, PSIO care is provided by the orthodontist, the pediatric dentist, or in some cases the patient's surgeon.

- PSIO treatment requires effort and dedication by the infant's caregivers; cooperation by attending all appointments and providing recommended home care is crucial for the best treatment outcome.

- Caregivers who have emergency concerns with the child's PSIO treatment should remove the appliance (if possible), examine the mouth and nose carefully, and contact the health care provider.

Presurgical infant orthopedics (PSIO) is a technique commonly used during the first months of life to prepare an infant with a cleft lip and palate for the first surgical repair. The aim of PSIO treatment is to reduce the size of the lip and alveolar clefts (gap in the gum pads) and in some cases alter the anatomy of the cleft-affected nose. This treatment lessens the severity of the cleft in preparation for the infant's primary surgical repair. Other names for PSIO include neonatal maxillary orthopedics, presurgical orthopedics, and maxillary orthopedics.

In the last 50 years, PSIO techniques have evolved with multiple variations. These techniques vary from simple lip taping to the use of more complex acrylic appliances for repositioning and reducing the width and severity of the cleft. According to a recent report, 71% of cleft centers in the United States and Canada use PSIO techniques. Nasoalveolar molding (NAM) was reported to be the most widely used PSIO method, with 55% of centers providing NAM therapy.

PRESURGICAL INFANT ORTHOPEDICS

History and Evolution

In the 1950s, McNeil popularized the first modern PSIO intraoral plate. A series of intraoral molding plates was used to reposition the alveolar segments. Hotz (1969) modified the plate to mold the alveolar segments into the normal anatomic position. Georgiade and Latham (1975) introduced an active pin-retained device to close the alveolar cleft or clefts. Nakajima (1990) described a splint for maintaining the nostril shape after the surgical cleft repair. Grayson (1993) introduced NAM. In addition to reducing the width of the cleft of the alveolar and lip segments, this technique also molds the nasal cartilage affected by the cleft.

Timing

The timing of PSIO treatment is critical; the tissues and cartilages of the nose and mouth are most easily molded during the infant's first 3 to 4 months of life possibly because of the presence in the baby's body of a maternal (from the child's mother) hormone called estrogen. Estrogen makes the baby's bones and cartilage flexible during delivery. The ease with which the mouth and nose can be molded gradu-

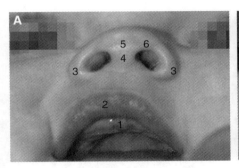

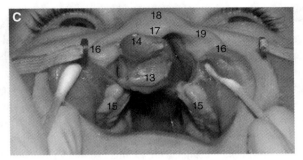

Fig. 27-1   A, Noncleft anatomy. **B,** Unilateral cleft lip and palate. **C,** Bilateral cleft lip and palate. (*1,* Alveolus. *2,* Upper lip. *3,* Alar base. *4,* Columella. *5,* Nasal tip. *6,* Nostril apex and alar rim. *7,* Greater alveolar segment. *8,* Lesser alveolar segment. *9,* Widened alar base. *10,* Deviated columella. *11,* Flattened nasal tip. *12,* Lateralized nostril apex and flattened alar rim. *13,* Protrusive premaxilla. *14,* Prolabium. *15,* Lateral alveolar segments. *16,* Widened alar base. *17,* Short or absent columella. *18,* Flat nasal tip. *19,* Lateralized nostril apex and flattened alar rim.)

ally decreases during the first months of the infant's life as maternal estrogen levels decrease; therefore the baby needs to be evaluated for possible PSIO treatment as soon as possible after birth. If the baby is diagnosed with a cleft on a prenatal ultrasound evaluation, the parents should contact the nearest cleft center to discuss treatment options and to prepare before the baby's birth (see Chapter 6).

Cleft anatomy is variable from patient to patient, because every infant is unique. A cleft affecting one side is called a unilateral cleft, whereas a cleft affecting both sides is called a bilateral cleft (Fig. 27-1). The cleft can affect only the lip, only the palate, or both. A cleft can affect the entire lip and extend into the nose (complete cleft lip) or only partially affect the lip (partial or incomplete cleft lip). In a cleft lip, a small band of tissue at the bottom of the nose called a *Simonart's band* may be present. The extent of palatal and alveolar clefting also ranges from complete to incomplete. The severity and degree of involvement of clefting vary considerably; approximately 240 possible combinations have been reported.

In patients with a unilateral cleft, the alveolar bone is divided into two components called the greater alveolar segment and the lesser alveolar segment, which are associated with the greater and lesser lip segments (see Fig. 27-1, *B*). Patients with a bilateral cleft have two lateral (side) alveolar segments (and associated lip segments) and a center part of the alveolus, called the *premaxilla* (see Fig. 27-1, *C*). The vomer (bottom part of the nasal septum, near the mouth) attaches behind and above the premaxilla. The lip segment in front of the premaxilla is called the *prolabium*.

In addition to altering the anatomy of the lip and mouth, the cleft also changes the nasal anatomy. The tip of the nose is flattened and loses its normal forward projection. The columella (strip of skin that separates the nostrils) is also affected. In patients with a unilateral cleft, the columella is deviated to one side. The columella is very deficient or absent in infants with a bilateral cleft. When viewed from below, the nostril apex (tip or area where the opening of the nostril is at the most convex point) is positioned to the side instead of forward. The *alar base* of the nose (side-to-side width where the nostril attaches to the lip) is also widened because of the cleft of the mouth and lips (see Figs. 27-1, *B* and *C*).

Benefits and Outcomes

The overall goal of PSIO is to normalize the cleft anatomy in preparation for the infant's primary lip and nose surgery. The reduced severity of the cleft optimizes the anatomy for the surgeon, and less tension is placed on the healing surgical site. Specifically, this is accomplished through the following PSIO goals:
- Reduction of the lip cleft
- Reduction of the alveolar cleft

In some PSIO techniques, the cleft nasal anatomy is addressed. The goals of treatment are the following:
- Increased columellar length and normalized columellar orientation
- Reduction of the alar base width
- Redirection of the nostril apex from a lateral position to an anterior (forward) position
- Increased nasal tip projection

Techniques

Many PSIO techniques are available. Parents should consult their cleft center to learn which, if any, PSIO options are offered and to understand the treatment alter-

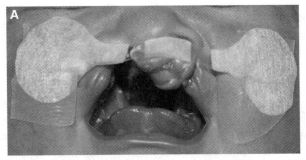

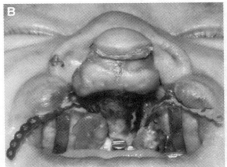

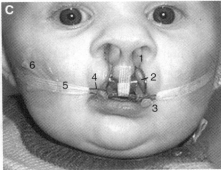

Fig. 27-2   **A,** Lip taping with DynaCleft tape. **B,** Latham device. **C,** NAM appliance. (*1,* Nasal stent. *2,* Wire holding the nasal stent to the mouth plate. *3,* Retention button. *4,* Orthodontic elastic, stretched to activate the appliance. *5,* Steri-Strip tape. *6,* Base tape.)

natives. The cleft care team will provide guidance regarding the best available options for the infant's cleft anatomy, the resources and techniques available through the center, and resources for the parents and other caregivers regarding timing of treatments, transportation to appointments, and any other family priorities. Each PSIO technique has benefits and limitations. The PSIO techniques discussed in this chapter are lip taping, the *Latham device,* and NAM (Fig. 27-2).

Lip Taping

Lip taping involves taping the cleft lip segments together, creating a tension that closes the gap in the lip and alveolar segments. One taping method to approximate the soft tissues of the lip, nose, and maxilla before primary cleft lip repair uses a surgical tape (sometimes with a small elastic incorporated into the tape) that is stretched over the lip segments. A commercially available taping system called DynaCleft (Canica Design, Inc., Barrie, Ontario, Canada) is commonly used in many centers (see Fig. 27-2, *A*).

Advantages
- Lip taping is easy to use.
- The need for follow-up visits to the cleft center is minimal.
- It is compatible in conjunction with and/or before the initiation of other PSIO techniques.
- It is relatively inexpensive.

Disadvantages
- The position of the alveolar segments is not fully controlled; the segments may move into an undesirable position relative to each other and to the surrounding anatomy.
- Lip taping does not address the nasal anatomy affected by the cleft.

Basic Steps for Effective Lip Taping
- The cheek and lip areas are cleaned before taping.
- The lip segments are manually brought together, closing the cleft.
- The tape is gently stretched and applied to the lip segments.
- Full-time lip taping (24 hours a day) is recommended for the best outcome.
- The lip tape can be replaced when soiled and when the adhesive is no longer sticky.

Latham Appliance

For patients with a unilateral cleft lip and palate, the Latham appliance is composed of two acrylic plates that fit over the alveolar segments. These plates are held in place on the alveolar segments by small pins that extend through the appliance and into the alveolus. The plates are connected by a hinged bar. A screw in the area of the cleft advances and expands the lesser segment of the unilateral cleft and retracts the greater segment backward and toward the midline; this screw is activated (turned) daily for 3 to 4 weeks. In patients with bilateral clefting, the Latham appliance retracts the premaxilla through the use of an elastic chain and expands the lateral alveolar segments with an activated expansion device. The patient is seen weekly for 4 to 7 weeks to activate the elastic chain. The expansion device is either activated during these visits, or at home by the caregiver. The cleft surgery takes place when the child is approximately 3 to 4 months of age (see Fig. 27-2, *B*).

Advantages
- With a Latham appliance, the alveolar segments close relatively quickly.
- The adjustment appointments are short.
- No extraoral taping is needed. The Latham appliance is an intraoral device, with no significant extraoral component.

Disadvantages

- Attachment of the appliance requires an additional surgical procedure in which the child is under general anesthesia; risks associated with surgery apply.
- The nasal anatomy affected by the cleft is not treated.

Latham Treatment and Adjustment Sequence

- An impression of the infant's mouth is made.
- The acrylic appliance is fabricated based on a stone model made from the mouth impression.
- The device is attached to the alveolus in the operating room while the child is under general anesthesia.
- The appliance is adjusted at regular intervals, as determined by the treating doctor.
- The appliance is removed at the time of the patient's primary surgical repair.

Nasoalveolar Molding

NAM combines an intraoral orthopedic plate with a nasal stent—the intraoral, extraoral, and nasal anatomy affected by the cleft are treated with this technique. The removable intraoral mouth plate is made of acrylic, which is similar to the material used for orthodontic retainers. After the patient attends a series of adjustment appointments to close the alveolar gap, the nasal stent (wire foundation with hard and soft acrylic covering) is attached to the extraoral button (Fig. 27-3, *A*). In general, the alveolar gap or gaps are closed to approximately 5 mm before the nasal stent is placed. The NAM provider adjusts the intraoral component and the nasal stent weekly or every other week (Fig. 27-4; see also Figs. 27-2, *C*, and 27-3).

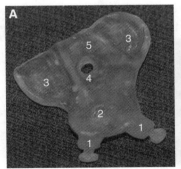
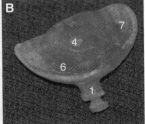

Fig. 27-3   A, Bilateral cleft NAM plate component. **B,** Unilateral cleft NAM plate components. (*1,* Retention buttons. *2,* Premaxilla. *3,* Lateral alveolar process. *4,* Airway hole. *5,* Vomer area. *6,* Greater alveolar segment. *7,* Lesser alveolar segment.)

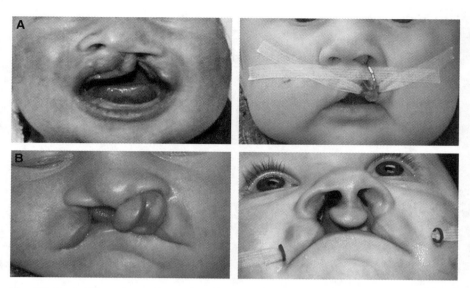

Fig. 27-4   A, This patient with a unilateral cleft lip and palate is shown before *(left)* and midway through treatment with a NAM device *(right).* **B,** This patient with a bilateral cleft lip and palate is shown before *(left)* and after treatment with a NAM device *(right).*

Advantages

- The alveolar segments are molded into a more normal position, reducing the alveolar cleft.
- The lip segments are brought together, reducing the size of the lip gap.
- The nasal differences are treated. (The nasal tip projection is less flat, the alar base width is reduced, the nostril apex is in a more forward location and will continue to grow in this direction instead of to the side, and the columella is lengthened and reoriented.)

Disadvantages

- Treatment using NAM is time consuming.
- An adjustment is needed weekly or every other week for 3 to 6 months, depending on the severity of the cleft.

Steps for Appliance Fabrication and Adjustment Sequence

- A dental impression is made of the maxilla and nose using a nontearing silicon material.

- An acrylic appliance based on the model of the infant's mouth is made in the dental laboratory.
- A base tape (wide tape that stays in place for 2 to 3 days to protect the infant's skin) is applied to the infant's cheek. A surgical tape and elastic (attached to the extraoral button on the NAM appliance) is applied to the base tape. This retains the molding plate in the mouth.
- The molding plate is modified weekly or every other week to guide the alveolar cleft segments into the desired position. Adjustments are made for 3 to 4 months for patients with a unilateral cleft and approximately 6 months in bilateral cleft patients.
- When the intraoral cleft or clefts are reduced to approximately 5 mm, the nasal stent is added to the mouth plate.
- The nasal stent and intraoral component are adjusted gradually during each appointment.
- Lip taping (prolabium taping or horizontal taping to the lip segments) may be used to help approximate the lip segments.

Care of the Nasoalveolar Molding Appliance

Nasoalveolar molding appliances retain milk and mouth and nasal secretions; therefore they require regular cleaning. After every feeding, the device is removed and cleaned with warm water and a soft brush or warm washcloth. Boiling water and even hot water distort the shape of the appliance and should not be used. The baby's oral and nasal cavities also should be kept clean with a moistened washcloth to preserve healthy tissues during NAM therapy and in preparation for surgery. The appliance should be protected from pets.

Management of Nasoalveolar Molding Complications

Complications from NAM therapy are generally minor and can be managed by examination and communication with the provider. The most common difficulties with treatment are cheek and/or nasal tissue irritation from the appliance. If this occurs, parents should remove the appliance; examine the baby's mouth, nose, and the appliance carefully; and contact the NAM treatment provider. If possible, they should take a photograph of the area and electronically send it to the treatment provider. Knowledge about the infant's relevant anatomy, a careful examination, and an accurate description of the problem are essential for effective management. Compliance with instructions about wear and care of the appliance is critical for treatment success and prevention of problems. With proper care and regular follow-up visits with the treatment provider, NAM treatment has a low incidence of complications, and major complications are rare.

Although every scenario is unique and requires individualized assessment, the following general guidelines are helpful.

- The baby is crying inconsolably or will not feed with the appliance in place. The NAM provider should be contacted immediately for adjustment of the device.
- Intraoral/intranasal sores can be caused by rough or irregular spots on the appliance rubbing against the soft tissue. They are typically treated by appliance alteration and polishing by the NAM provider. If the ulceration is more significant, the provider may recommend adjustment of the appliance and temporary appliance removal until tissues are healed. Depending on the location of the tissue irritation, a moisturizing agent or salve may be indicated.
- Cheek irritation from taping is treated by changing the location of tape on the cheek and applying a moisturizer or salve to the cheek.
- Ectopic *neonatal teeth* (early eruption of teeth) may occur. The NAM plate can be modified to fit around the erupting tooth, or tooth removal may be indicated.
- Retention of the appliance may be a problem. The appliance might not fit, because it is wearing inconsistently, the plate or nasal stent requires adjustment, or the taping strength or angulation needs to be altered. If the infant dislodges the plate, parents can consider placing mitts on the baby's hands.
- If the appliance is broken or distorted, it should be removed from the infant's mouth and the provider should be contacted. Breakage could pose a risk of the infant inhaling or swallowing a piece of the appliance. If this is suspected or if breathing difficulties are noted, the infant should be taken to the nearest emergency department immediately for medical attention. The broken or distorted appliance can be fixed at the next NAM appointment or at an emergency visit if indicated.

FEEDING WITH PRESURGICAL INFANT ORTHOPEDIC APPLIANCES AND NASOALVEOLAR MOLDING

Most infants adapt to feeding with PSIO devices fairly easily. The cleft team feeding specialist will guide the parents during the initiation of PSIO treatment. Patients with a NAM appliance should be observed for changes in feeding pattern. This can occur if the device does not fit properly and causes discomfort. The appliance may require a special adjustment.

LIP ADHESION: SURGICAL ALTERNATIVE TO PRESURGICAL INFANT ORTHOPEDICS

Some cleft treatment centers perform a lip adhesion surgery before the definitive primary lip and nose surgery. A lip adhesion is a preliminary surgery in which the lips segments are attached, converting a complete cleft lip to an incomplete cleft lip. The tension placed on the lips also closes the alveolar cleft to facilitate the final surgical repair. The cleft lip adhesion surgery is performed around 2 months of age and nose surgery is performed when the baby is approximately 3 months of age and weighs at least 10 pounds.

Advantages

- The lip and alveolar segments are brought together, allowing closure of the definitive repair with less tension on the tissues.
- Weekly visits are not needed, as with some PSIO techniques.

Disadvantages

- Lip adhesion requires an additional surgical procedure in which the child is under general anesthesia; this bears the risks associated with surgery.
- The closed alveolar segments may be misaligned.
- The cleft nasal anatomy is not treated.

CONCLUSION

PSIO is a technique some cleft centers use to lessen the cleft severity in preparation for the infant's primary surgical repair. Numerous PSIO techniques are available; each has benefits and limitations. Parents should discuss options with the cleft center team coordinator, the surgeon, and the PSIO provider to determine the best treatment for their child.

28

Orthodontic Principles in the Management of Orofacial Clefts

Ana M. Mercado

KEY POINTS

- Orthodontia is a key part of the cleft treatment plan that helps to ensure proper function and appearance of the teeth and jaws.

- People with clefts can benefit from orthodontics in different ways throughout their cleft treatment plan, from infancy to the completion of growth.

- Orthodontic interventions are performed in stages; the timing depends on the patient's dental development and coordination with the rest of the cleft treatment plan.

- Surgery and orthodontia complement one another throughout the cleft treatment plan.

The timing and sequencing of orthodontic care requires prioritizing the patient's other health care needs in an integrated treatment plan that involves all team members. Orthodontic interventions are classified into four distinct periods defined by the patient's age and dental development: the neonatal period, the primary dentition period, the mixed dentition period, and the permanent dentition period (see Chapter 26). Orthodontic treatment is best delivered in separate stages, avoiding continuous treatment from the early mixed dentition to the permanent dentition.

NEONATAL MAXILLARY ORTHOPEDICS

Neonatal (infant) orthopedic treatment occurs during the first few postnatal months unless contraindicated by other congenital conditions that place the infant's health at risk. This intervention was introduced in the 1960s for the purpose of aligning the maxillary alveolar segments. The simplest form of infant orthopedics is lip taping (Fig. 28-1). This early intervention helps the surgeons by decreasing the gap between the lip segments (Table 28-1).

The technique of nasoalveolar molding (NAM) involves an intraoral molding plate, nasal stents, and extraoral taping (see Chapter 27). Intraorally, the alveolar ridges are molded to reduce the size of the cleft by approximating the segments. Extraorally, the use of nasal stents and taping lengthens the columella in patients with

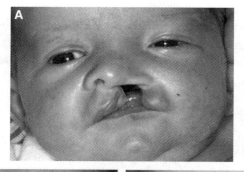

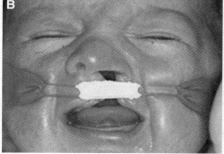
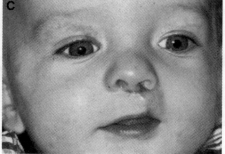

Fig. 28-1 This infant has a complete unilateral left cleft lip and palate. **A,** The cleft lip is shown before orthopedic treatment. **B,** Presurgical orthopedics with lip taping helps to approximate the segments before the surgical lip repair. **C,** The child is shown after the surgical lip repair.

a bilateral cleft lip and realigns the sides of the nose in bilateral and unilateral cleft lip patients. This orthopedic treatment prepares the infant for lip-nose surgical repair, sometimes in combination with a *gingival* surgery to close the alveolar defect.

If neonatal orthopedics is recommended and feasible, it is completed in the first few months after birth so that a definitive surgical lip repair can be performed before the child is 6 months of age. Palate repair is usually delayed until the infant is 12 to 18 months of age (see Chapter 23).

Table 28-1   Timeline for Dental and Orthodontic Treatment of Cleft Lip and Palate

Age Range	Intervention
Birth to 3 months	Evaluation and start of neonatal infant orthopedics
3 to 6 months	Continued infant orthopedics as needed
6 to 12 months	Start of pediatric dental care with the first dental visit, prevention of tooth decay, and restoration
4 to 6 years	Orthodontic evaluation for the need of palatal expansion and/or a protraction face mask (see Figs. 28-4 and 28-5)
7 to 11 years	Preparation for bone grafting, including palatal expansion and/or limited incisor alignment Alveolar bone grafting
12 to 15 years	After bone grafting, limited orthodontics with further palatal expansion and dental alignment Monitoring of jaw growth
16 to 18 years	Comprehensive orthodontics with or without jaw surgery Preparation of spaces for future replacement of missing teeth
18 to 21 years	Definitive restoration of missing teeth with dental implants and/or a fixed or removable prosthesis

This treatment timeline varies from child to child, depending on individual characteristics of the cleft, the developing dentition, the facial growth pattern, and the child's other health care needs.

PRIMARY DENTITION

The primary teeth have usually fully come in by the time the child is 2½ to 3 years of age. At this age, the facial soft tissues can mask an underlying skeletal deficiency (Figs. 28-2 and 28-3). As the toddler grows, the growth of the maxilla (upper jaw) lags behind the growth of the mandible (lower jaw), increasing the midface deficiency. This *retrusion* of the nose and cheeks relative to the lower jaw and chin

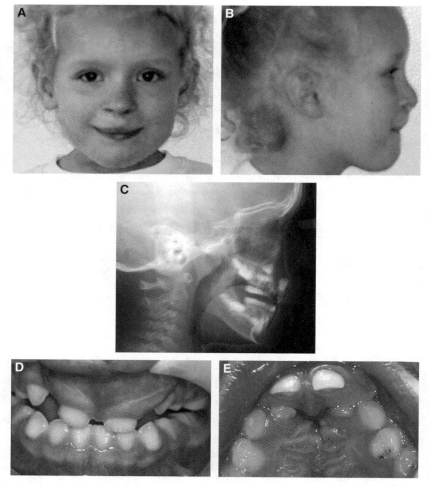

Fig. 28-2 **A,** This 6-year-old girl has a repaired complete bilateral cleft lip and palate. **B,** A profile view shows a mildly prominent maxilla. **C,** A lateral skull radiograph shows her primary dentition. **D,** An intraoral view shows the bilateral crossbite tendency. **E,** An intraoral view shows a fistula in the palate and the primary (baby) lateral incisors erupted behind the premaxilla.

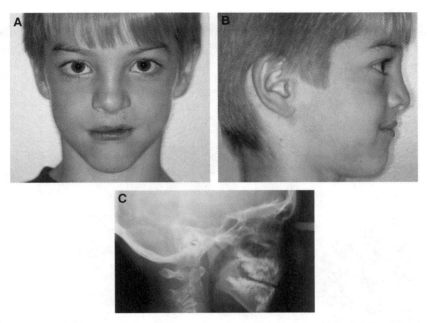

Fig. 28-3   A, This 7-year-old boy has a repaired complete unilateral left cleft lip and palate. **B,** A profile view shows mild retrusion of the maxilla and mandible. **C,** A lateral skull radiograph shows his early mixed dentition.

may result in an anterior crossbite and/or a *posterior crossbite*. In some children, a crossbite signals the need for orthodontic treatment in the primary dentition. Because the crossbite is likely to return when the permanent teeth come in, orthodontic treatment may be postponed until the mixed dentition period.

The treatment of early skeletal midface deficiency can be somewhat successful if therapy begins in the primary or early mixed dentition period with a protraction face mask (Figs. 28-4 and 28-5). This therapy consists of an intraoral appliance with hooks and an extraoral removable face mask that the patient wears at night. The patient wears elastics that extend from the intraoral hooks to a horizontal bar on the face mask. This force pulls the upper jaw forward. The upper jaw improvement may not be permanent. As the child grows, the growth of the maxilla continues to lag behind the normal mandibular growth. Consequently, the malocclusion reestablishes during the late mixed dentition period and into the adolescent permanent dentition period. When indicated, the most logical time for the intervention is before the child is 10 years of age, at which time the sutures between the facial bones are more responsive to force. However, a severe malocclusion in the primary or early mixed dentition is unlikely to be corrected with a protraction face mask. In such severe malocclusions, skeletal correction should be delayed until the permanent dentition stage.

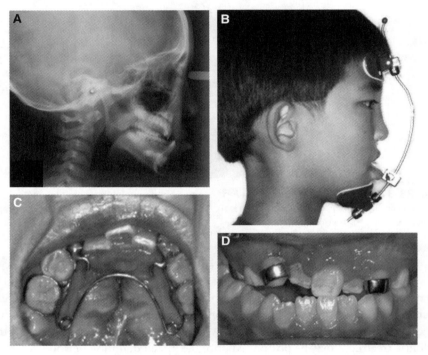

Fig. 28-4   This 8-year-old boy has a repaired complete unilateral right cleft lip and palate with a maxillary deficiency. **A,** A lateral skull radiograph shows an anterior crossbite. **B,** He wears a protraction face mask with elastics attached to hooks on an expander. **C,** His palatal expander has bands cemented on his maxillary primary molars and canines, with palatal hooks to attach elastics. **D,** His posterior and anterior crossbites are improving with palatal expansion and maxillary and dental protraction.

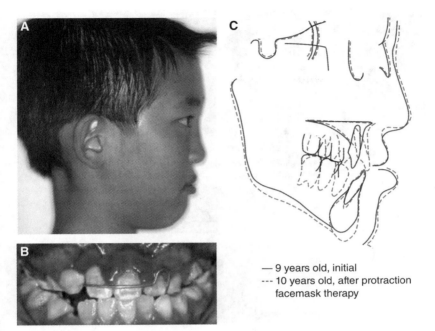

— 9 years old, initial
--- 10 years old, after protraction
    facemask therapy

Fig. 28-5   A, This patient, who is also in Fig. 28-4, is shown after 9 months of protraction face mask therapy and palatal expansion. **B,** An intraoral view shows correction of his anterior and posterior crossbites. The maxillary retainer is in place. **C,** Superimposition of the initial tracings from *cephalometric radiographs* and those obtained after protraction therapy show correction of his anterior crossbite by incisor *proclination* and mild maxillary advancement.

MIXED DENTITION

The dental development undergoes a transition when the child is 6 to 12 years of age. The primary teeth are lost, and the permanent teeth come in. The midface deficiency makes the mandible appear prominent, especially on a profile view (Fig. 28-6). Eruption of the permanent teeth coincides with a period of psychological transition during preadolescence when the sense of friendship intensifies and independence from parents increases. This is also the period when the greatest advances can be made in restoring the bone in the cleft site with alveolar bone grafts.

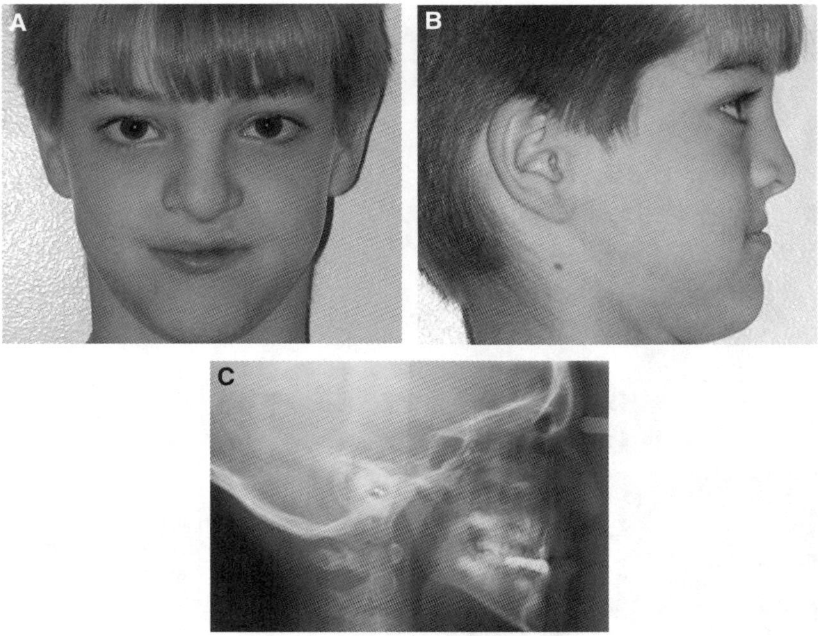

Fig. 28-6   **A,** This patient, who is shown in Fig. 28-3, is 9 years of age. **B,** A profile view shows mild midface deficiency. **C,** A lateral skull radiograph in the mixed dentition stage shows an anterior crossbite.

ALVEOLAR BONE GRAFTING

Primary Bone Grafting

Primary bone grafting typically involves placing a bone graft before eruption of the primary incisors at the time of the primary surgical lip repair. Most cleft palate teams prefer to wait until further maxillary growth and development has occurred. This is known as secondary bone grafting.

Secondary Bone Grafting

Secondary alveolar bone grafting is classified according to the patient age at which the bone graft is placed: early secondary bone grafting (2 to 5 years of age), intermediate or secondary bone grafting (6 to 15 years of age), or late secondary bone grafting (adolescence to adulthood).

Currently grafting is thought to be most appropriate during the intermediate period (6 to 15 years of age), because it does not interfere with maxillary growth and provides bone at the cleft site before the adjacent teeth erupt. A survey of teams across North America revealed that most of the centers perform intermediate alveolar bone grafting. Therefore the following discussion will focus on intermediate or secondary alveolar bone grafting.

Benefits of Secondary Alveolar Bone Grafting

Secondary alveolar bone grafting has several benefits, including the following:
- Placement of bone for eruption of the teeth at the cleft: A bone graft placed before eruption of the teeth that belong in the cleft (especially the maxillary lateral incisor and canine) facilitates the eruption of these teeth into a continuous alveolar ridge, bringing additional alveolar bone into the area (Fig. 28-7).
- Placement of bone for the teeth adjacent to the cleft: Teeth directly adjacent to the cleft, particularly maxillary central incisors, erupt into unfavorable positions, often tipped or rotated. Radiographs of these teeth show a thin layer of bone along their root (see Fig. 28-7). If the tipped teeth are aligned with orthodontic treatment, the thin layer of bone may dissolve, leaving the teeth with poor support and at risk of loss. If a bone graft is placed before extensive orthodontic alignment of erupted teeth adjacent to the cleft, the bone supporting the teeth is preserved, and orthodontic alignment after grafting can be accomplished with minimal risk of dissolving the preexisting bone.

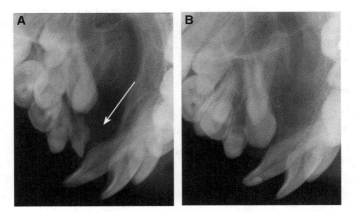

Fig. 28-7   A, This radiograph shows a bone defect *(arrow)* at the cleft site before alveolar bone grafting. The maxillary canine has more than two thirds of the root developed (close to eruption). A thin layer of bone covers the adjacent central incisor. No orthodontic incisor alignment is planned. **B,** This radiograph, taken 4 months after alveolar bone grafting, shows excellent fill of the cleft defect with bone. The canine is erupting through the grafted bone.

- Closure of oronasal fistulas: *Oronasal fistulas* can influence speech in patients with cleft lip and palate. Surgical closure of oronasal fistulas with secondary bone grafting results in a significant improvement of speech.
- Improvement in the shape and support of the nose: This benefit contributes to improved nasal and lip symmetry and provides a stable bone platform on which the nasal structures are supported.
- Reestablishment of continuity to the maxillary alveolar ridge: After a successful bone graft, the orthodontist can move the teeth safely into the cleft site. Dental implants can be placed into the grafted bone at the appropriate age to replace missing teeth.
- Stabilization of the maxillary segments: Patients with bilateral clefts have mobility of the premaxilla. In such cases, secondary bone grafting stabilizes the premaxilla.

Timing of Secondary Bone Grafting

The time for performing secondary alveolar bone grafting is based on either the patient's chronologic age or dental development.

Chronologic Age

By definition, secondary bone grafting is done in the mixed dentition before the eruption of the maxillary canine (or lateral incisor, if present). Therefore the graft needs to be performed before the eruption of the permanent teeth adjacent to the cleft, typically when the child is 6 to 15 years of age. The older the patient at the time of surgery, the poorer the results of secondary bone grafting. However, using chronologic age alone for defining the ideal age for grafting may not be useful, because patients with a cleft lip and/or palate have delayed development of the teeth, compared with those with no clefts. The child's dental development can be a more accurate indicator of the ideal timing for bone grafting.

Dental Development

The root formation of the permanent maxillary canine on the cleft side can be used as a developmental indicator for determining ideal timing of an alveolar graft. The recommended time is when the maxillary canine has developed half to two thirds of its final length, which generally occurs from 8 to 11 years of age (see Fig. 28-7). When the root has developed two thirds of its expected full length, the canine erupts rapidly. Eruption continues spontaneously through the graft, bringing additional alveolar bone into the area. When the maxillary lateral incisor is present and located posterior to (behind) the cleft, it may be advisable to graft before the eruption of the lateral incisor.

Sequencing

The sequencing of procedures for an alveolar bone graft requires interdisciplinary communication and cooperation for a successful result. Parents may be concerned about teeth (often extra teeth) that have erupted near the cleft either in the palate or directly under the lip. The cleaning of these *ectopic teeth* can be challenging for the parents and the patient. The general or pediatric dentist ensures that the patient and parents are aware of the ectopic teeth and provides instructions for good brushing practices to prevent decay. These teeth need to be preserved before surgery, because they maintain the supporting alveolus. Decayed teeth adjacent to the cleft should be restored before the grafting procedure. Erupted teeth adjacent to the cleft that are in poor condition should be extracted at least 2 months before surgery. This allows time for the soft tissues to heal (Fig. 28-8). Healthy ectopic primary or extra teeth that have erupted along the line of the cleft should also be removed at least 2 months before surgery. Orthodontic treatment may be required preoperatively to reposition maxillary teeth or to expand a narrow maxilla, thus providing the surgeon better access to the cleft defect. In patients with bilateral clefts, the mobile premaxilla may need to be protected from biting forces during the healing period, because such forces may compromise the success of the grafts. Other procedures such as minor aesthetic surgeries of the nose and lip and the insertion of ear tubes can be done at the time of the alveolar bone grafting procedure. Unerupted teeth adjacent to the cleft that have a poor prognosis can be removed at the time of surgery.

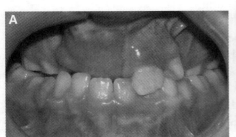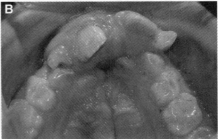

Fig. 28-8   This 7-year-old boy with a repaired complete bilateral cleft lip and palate is shown before alveolar bone grafting. **A,** An intraoral view shows an anterior crossbite, bilateral posterior crossbites, and a rotated incisor. **B,** Another intraoral view shows a narrow posterior maxillary arch, an oronasal fistula, a prominent premaxilla, extra lateral incisors in the palate, and decayed primary incisors. He needs maxillary expansion before bone grafting to improve the alignment of the narrow posterior maxillary arch with the premaxilla, selected extractions, and restorative care.

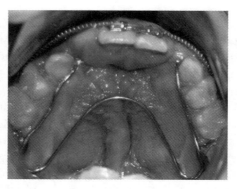

Fig. 28-9   This patient, who is presented in Fig. 28-8, is shown at 10 years of age, after maxillary expansion with a W arch, successful alveolar bone grafting, and incisor alignment.

Transverse Dimension (Dental Arch Width)

A maxillary expansion appliance such as a quad helix or a W arch, is often recommended to improve the alignment of the maxillary segments before an alveolar graft is placed (Fig. 28-9; see Fig. 28-8). The orthodontist will consult the surgeon about this procedure to prevent overexpansion of the maxillary arch and to preserve adequate soft tissue to close the site. Overexpansion of the dental arch can increase the width of the alveolar cleft and the size of the oronasal fistula. If the oronasal fistula is large, the surgeon may prefer to close it, allow the tissues to heal, and then proceed with alveolar bone grafting.

When maxillary expansion is needed before alveolar bone grafting, a quad helix or W-arch appliance is cemented with bands to the first permanent molars. The fixed appliance has lateral wire arms that extend anteriorly (forward) and can be adjusted. These appliances are easy to clean and provide a slow and continuous expanding force. After bone grafting and if more expansion is needed in the young permanent dentition, a maxillary expander with a palatal jackscrew can be used (Fig. 28-10).

Incisor Alignment

The incisors adjacent to the cleft are typically rotated and tipped because of the limited amount of bone covering their roots. Often, this malposition results in

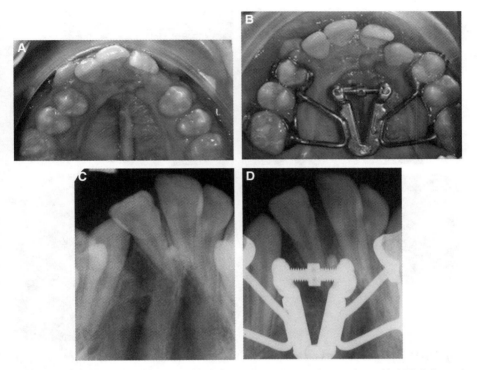

Fig. 28-10   A, This 10-year-old patient with a repaired complete unilateral left cleft lip and palate is shown after alveolar bone grafting and before maxillary (palatal) expansion. The premolar regions are narrow. **B,** The maxillary (palatal) expander is in place. A midline space is present between the maxillary central incisors. **C,** A radiograph taken before expansion shows excellent bony fill of the left alveolar cleft. **D,** A radiograph obtained during maxillary expansion shows the space between maxillary central incisors and evidence of an intact grafted area.

traumatic occlusion (a condition in which the edges of the upper and lower teeth strike one another) and limited access for the surgeon. In such cases, some degree of orthodontic alignment of the teeth may be needed. Orthodontic alignment of incisors before grafting is limited by the available bone into which the teeth can be moved.

After successful healing of the graft is confirmed on radiographs, teeth adjacent to the cleft can be moved (Fig. 28-11). Alignment of incisors shortly after successful healing of the bone graft contributes to better oral hygiene and improved self-esteem for the patient.

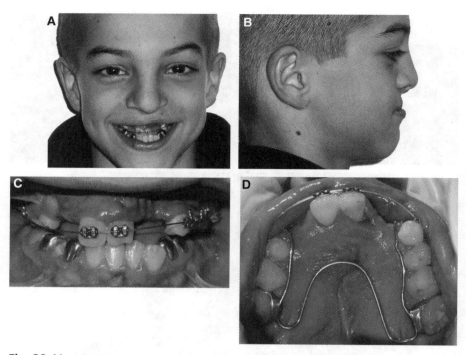

Fig. 28-11   A, This patient was presented in Figs. 28-3 and 28-6. He is shown at 11 years of age after successful alveolar bone grafting and is undergoing orthodontic treatment of his maxillary arch. **B,** A profile view shows more marked midface deficiency. **C,** An intraoral view shows limited orthodontic appliances, correction of anterior and posterior crossbites, and alignment of the incisors. **D,** A maxillary occlusal view shows a W arch in place and improved arch form.

Eruption of the Maxillary Canine

The maxillary canine erupts through the grafted bone (see Fig. 28-7) after surgery. The goal of orthodontic movement of the teeth is to create enough space in the arch for the canines to erupt after bone grafting. Often, the canine will erupt spontaneously after the bone graft. In the late mixed dentition and when more than two thirds of the root length has developed, a canine that does not show signs of spontaneous eruption over a reasonable period of time (4 to 6 months) will need to be surgically uncovered. This will facilitate its eruption into the arch, with or without orthodontic force.

Absence of the Maxillary Lateral Incisor

Numerous studies have shown that many patients with a cleft lip and palate have congenitally missing lateral incisors. Even when the lateral incisors are present, they may need to be extracted early in patients with nonrestorable decay, severe tooth malformations, or poor bone support. Therefore many children reach the age of secondary bone grafting without the maxillary lateral incisor next to the cleft.

In these patients, the canine is allowed to erupt next to the central incisors after bone grafting. The canine brings more alveolar bone into the area, thus preserving the width of the alveolar ridge. The orthodontic closure of the missing lateral space is usually referred to as *canine substitution,* because the maxillary canine is placed in the position of the lateral incisor. The other option is to preserve the missing lateral space for a future dental implant with a prosthetic crown.

Assessing the Outcome of Secondary Bone Grafting

The success or failure of an alveolar bone graft requires an evaluation of the bone in the cleft and the bone covering the adjacent teeth and those migrating into the cleft. Current methods include conventional radiography and cone-beam computed tomography (CBCT).

Radiographic Appearance of the Bone

Intraoral radiographs are typically used for assessing the quality of alveolar bone grafts. However, one limitation of this technique is that a radiograph produces a two-dimensional representation of a three-dimensional area (the cleft). Some structures of interest will not be clearly visible, because adjacent structures block them. Nevertheless, the use of dental radiographs is considered a standard of care, because it is a relatively noninvasive, efficient, and economical method.

Cone-Beam Computed Tomography

Cone-beam computed tomography shows the bone graft in three dimensions. The size of the defect and the position of the teeth next to the cleft can be assessed more accurately than with conventional radiographs. This information is valuable for diagnostic assessment before orthodontic movement of adjacent teeth into the cleft, eruption of a canine through the graft, or insertion of dental implants in the grafted area.

PERMANENT DENTITION

The permanent dentition is established with the eruption of the canines and premolars. Generally, the eruption of the young permanent dentition coincides with the body changes of puberty. Noticeable characteristics include facial hair and voice changes in males and breast development in females. A growth spurt occurs, characterized by an acceleration followed by a deceleration in height gain. Growth of the skull and face includes an increase in mandibular growth that causes a worsening in facial appearance and occlusion (Figs. 28-12 through 28-14). Self-consciousness is normal during adolescence, but it may become more intense when a teen has a visible facial difference.

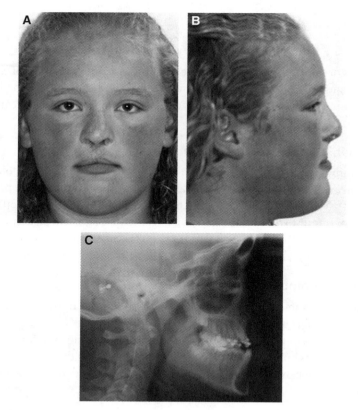

Fig. 28-12   A, This patient is also shown in Fig. 28-2. She is 15 years of age. Alveolar bone grafting is completed, and she is undergoing limited orthodontic alignment. **B,** She has a concave facial profile and a midface deficiency. **C,** A lateral skull radiograph shows maxillary retrusion, proclined maxillary incisors, and an anterior crossbite. The need for jaw surgery (forward movement of the upper jaw) is apparent.

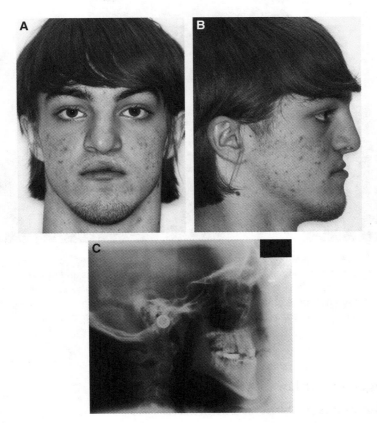

Fig. 28-13   A, This patient is shown in Figs. 28-3, 28-6, and 28-11. He is 16 years of age and interested in combined orthodontic-surgical treatment and future dental implants. **B,** A profile view shows retrusion in both jaws, especially in the maxilla, and a concave facial profile. **C,** A lateral skull radiograph shows retrusion in both jaws and an anterior crossbite.

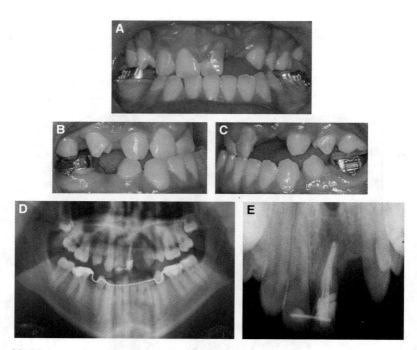

Fig. 28-14   **A-C,** This patient is shown in Figs. 28-3, 28-6, 28-11, and 28-13. He is shown at 6 years of age with an anterior crossbite with backward tipped incisors and signs of insufficient gum tissue. The lower lingual holding arch is in place. **D,** A *panoramic radiograph* shows several congenitally missing teeth and evidence of endodontic treatment and a large composite restoration on the maxillary left central incisor. **E,** Bone fill is adequate at the cleft site.

Management of Jaw Discrepancies

Considerations for Skeletal-Facial Aesthetics

Patients with unilateral complete clefts of the lip and palate typically become more maxillary deficient, and their mandibles appear more prominent as they reach adolescence and adulthood. This is from a deficiency in maxillary growth resulting in a concave facial profile (see Figs. 28-12 and 28-13).

Patients with mild skeletal discrepancies and minimal aesthetic concerns may benefit from treatment by orthodontics alone (Figs. 28-15 and 28-16). A change in the slant of the teeth (moving the maxillary incisors forward and/or moving the mandibular incisors backward), selective extractions, shaving the sides of the teeth, and/or cosmetic bonding may adequately mask the skeletal discrepancy. However, children in whom such dental compensations are performed before growth has stabilized may outgrow the correction, and jaw surgery may be recommended later.

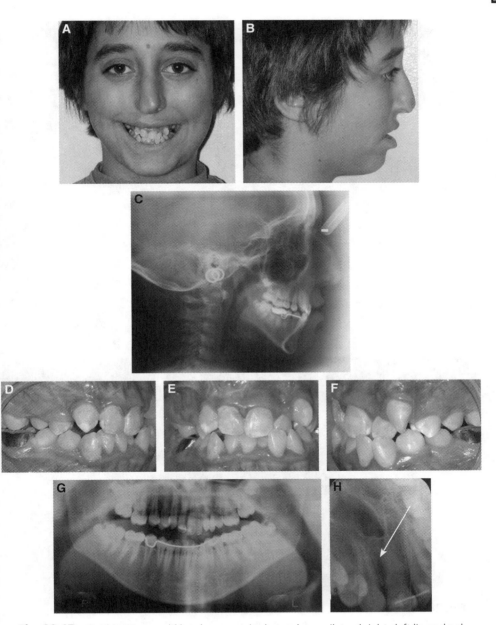

Fig. 28-15   A, This 13-year-old boy has a repaired complete unilateral right cleft lip and palate. He is interested in orthodontic treatment without jaw surgery. **B,** A profile view shows retrusion in both jaws and a mildly convex facial profile. **C,** A lateral skull radiograph shows retrusion in both jaws and upright incisors. **D-F,** Intraoral views show severe crowding in both arches and significant midline deviation. The lower lingual holding arch is in place. **G,** A panoramic radiograph shows that a maxillary right lateral incisor was removed previously. It was malformed and without root development. **H,** A radiograph shows adequate alveolar bone fill at the cleft site *(arrow).*

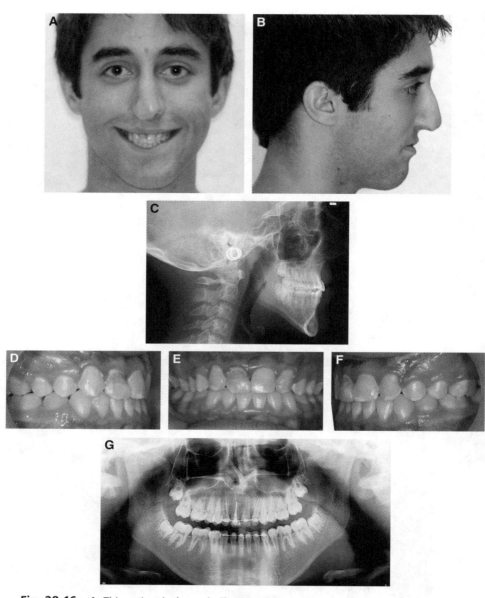

Fig. 28-16   **A,** This patient is shown in Fig. 28-15. He is 17 years of age and has completed orthodontic treatment (nonsurgical). **B,** A profile view shows retrusion in both jaws and a mildly convex profile. **C,** A lateral skull radiograph shows retrusion in both jaws, proclination of the upper incisors, and *retroclination* of the lower incisors. **D-F,** Intraoral views. The orthodontic plan included extraction of several teeth, a maxillary expander, and maxillary canine substitution on both sides. **G,** A panoramic radiograph shows evidence of root canal treatment in the maxillary right lateral incisor and permanent bonded retainers.

Patients with severe skeletal discrepancies and significant aesthetic concerns are candidates for orthodontic treatment combined with jaw surgery (see Figs. 28-12 and 28-13). Conventional surgical correction of severe maxillary deficiency (greater than 10 mm) commonly involves the advancement of the maxilla as much as possible within the constraints of the scar tissue from the lip and palate repairs.

The amount of maxillary advancement is often not sufficient to correct the skeletal discrepancy. Simultaneous surgical setback (backward movement) of the mandible may be done to correct the remaining skeletal discrepancy. The disadvantage of this two-jaw approach in patients with clefts is that facial balance may be compromised by setting the mandible back.

Orthognathic Surgery

Timing and Sequencing

In patients with severe skeletal discrepancies, deciding to delay surgical orthodontic treatment until growth is complete may be sound judgment for a more stable result. Cephalometric radiographs obtained once or twice a year can be superimposed to identify this postpubertal period of slow facial growth. Comprehensive treatment, including extractions, orthodontics, and jaw surgery, should be delayed until after the pubertal growth spurt has occurred. Lip and nose surgical revisions are typically postponed until after jaw surgery and prosthetic rehabilitation of the dentition are complete.

Role of the Orthodontist

The presurgical phase of orthodontic treatment lasts about 12 to 18 months. The goals are to align the teeth, coordinate the dental arches, and distribute space for prosthetic teeth. This may cause the malocclusion to look worse as the teeth are placed in their correct relationship to the underlying skeletal bases (Fig. 28-17). After these goals are met, the patient is referred to the surgeon for a consultation. Once the orthodontist and the surgeon agree that the presurgical setup is acceptable, the orthodontist places full-size intraoral arch wires with crimped or soldered lugs to provide a means for fixating the maxilla and/or mandible into the proper occlusion immediately after surgery.

After surgical correction of the jaw discrepancy, the upper and lower teeth should fit together well. During the postsurgical period, the surgeon continues to manage the patient for several weeks to ensure that no complications occur during the healing phase. Once the patient is stable and can tolerate a soft diet, the postsurgical phase of orthodontics treatment can proceed. In this phase, which should be completed within 4 to 6 months, the occlusion is fine-tuned, and the preparations are finalized for the replacement of missing teeth (Figs. 28-18 and 28-19).

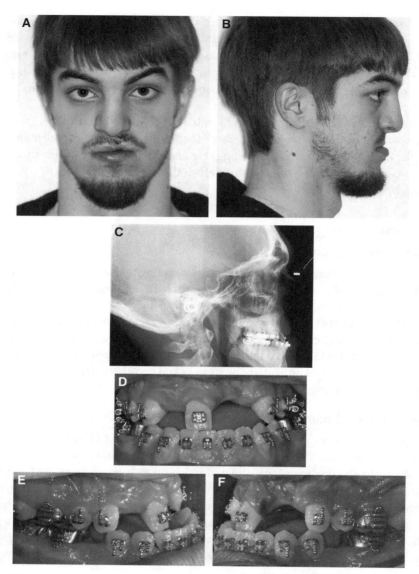

Fig. 28-17   **A,** This patient is shown in Figs. 28-3, 28-6, 28-11, 28-13, and 28-14. He is 19 years of age and has completed presurgical orthodontic treatment. He has chosen a single-jaw surgery. **B,** A profile view shows a more accentuated concave facial profile. **C,** A lateral skull radiograph shows more proclined maxillary and mandibular incisors. **D-F,** Intraoral views show an anterior crossbite. The maxillary left central incisor was extracted because of increased bone loss and mobility. Gingival grafting was done on the lower incisor region before incisor alignment.

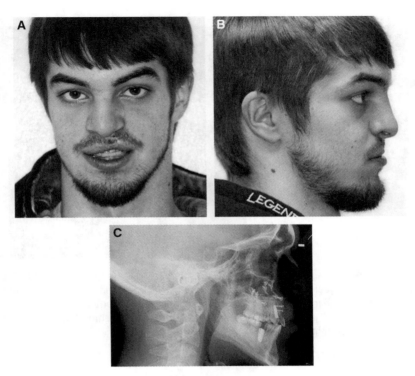

Fig. 28-18   A, This patient is shown in Figs. 28-3, 28-6, 28-11, 28-13, 28-14, and 28-17. He is 20 years of age and has had maxillary advancement surgery. **B,** He has a more balanced facial profile. **C,** A lateral skull radiograph shows improved maxillary positioning. Dental implants have been placed. Miniscrews have been placed to hold a bone graft, increasing the bone level in the anterior maxilla.

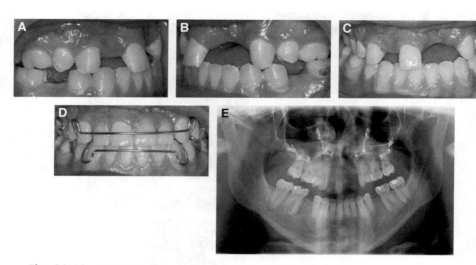

Fig. 28-19 **A-C,** This patient is shown in Figs. 28-3, 28-6, 28-11, 28-13, 28-14, 28-17, and 28-18. He is 20 years of age and has completed jaw surgery. His occlusion is adequate. **D,** *Hawley retainers* are in place. The maxillary retainer has pontics for temporary replacement of missing incisors. **E,** A panoramic radiograph was obtained after removal of the braces and before implant placement.

On removal of orthodontic appliances, fixed retainers in the form of a wire bonded to the back of the incisors are used to maintain the alignment of the incisors. However, the previously corrected crossbite of the posterior teeth can recur (if tooth position is not retained) after the arch wires are removed. A maxillary acrylic plate or a Hawley retainer may be recommended to hold the posterior teeth in the correct position and for prosthetic replacement of missing teeth (see Fig. 28-19, *C* and *D*).

Distraction Osteogenesis

With *distraction osteogenesis* it may be possible to correct a severely deficient maxilla by forward advancement alone (Fig. 28-20). With this technique, the extent of maxillary advancement can be greater than the 10 mm possible with conventional jaw surgery. This is accomplished by gradual traction of the mobilized maxilla and the palatal tissues during the slow distraction over time.

The technique of rigid external distraction involves cementation of an appliance on the maxillary teeth, with metal hooks extending out of the mouth for traction. In surgery, cuts are made on the maxilla, and a rigid external distraction device (which acts as a bone anchor) is attached to the immobile part of the skull (Fig. 28-21). Patients perform the distraction at home by turning a screw at a rate of

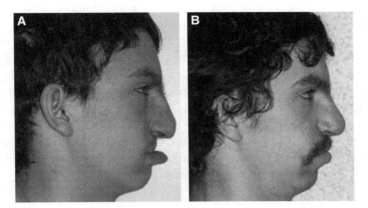

Fig. 28-20   A, This 17-year-old male has a repaired complete bilateral cleft lip and palate. He has retrusion of both jaws and severe maxillary deficiency. **B,** He is shown after advancement of the maxilla with distraction osteogenesis with an improved maxilla position. The patient may benefit from mandibular advancement surgery.

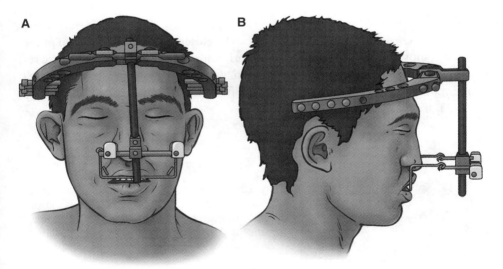

Fig. 28-21   Rigid external distraction device.

1 mm per day; this moves the maxilla forward relative to the immobile part of the skull. After the desired advancement is achieved, the device is left in place for 2 to 3 weeks to allow bone consolidation. A retention period follows during which the patient wears a removable protraction face mask.

Some patients treated with distraction osteogenesis will still require additional surgical procedures for the maxilla and/or mandible in the postadolescent period. The orthodontist and the oral surgeon should counsel patients and their families presurgically on the possible need for additional surgery (see Fig. 28-20).

One benefit of distraction osteogenesis is that, with gradual advancement of the palate in small increments, the soft palate and pharynx have time to adapt. In addition, hypernasal speech can be monitored (see Chapter 12).

Management of the Missing Lateral Incisor Space

In patients with missing teeth in the region of the cleft, several options are available for the management of the space. The most common options include space closure, a fixed or removable prosthesis, and dental implants.

Space Closure

The space created by the missing tooth can be closed by allowing eruption of the canine, moving the posterior teeth anteriorly with orthodontics, and cosmetic reshaping of the canine. This approach eliminates the need for a prosthetic replacement of the absent lateral incisor and is often called a canine substitution (Fig. 28-22; see Fig. 28-16, *E*).

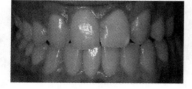

Fig. 28-22 This 18-year-old male with a repaired complete unilateral left cleft lip and palate is shown after completion of combined surgical-orthodontic treatment. After bilateral maxillary canine substitution, canines should be reshaped to resemble lateral incisors.

Fixed and Removable Prosthesis

Fixed prostheses are recommended for nongrowing patients with a single tooth missing in the cleft area, patients who need permanent stabilization of the maxillary segments (cases of failed or nonexistent alveolar bone grafts), and patients whose adjacent teeth are malformed and could benefit from crowns. On the other hand, removable prostheses are indicated for replacing multiple teeth along the arch, for obturation (plugging) of large palatal fistulas, for adding acrylic to improve lip support in patients with severe alveolar defects, and for temporary replacement of teeth in young patients.

Osseointegrated Dental Implants

It is possible to replace missing teeth in the cleft area with dental implants. This is performed to restore a single missing tooth, without the need to reduce healthy enamel on adjacent teeth. It is also performed to stabilize fixed or removable dentures. An adequate volume of alveolar bone at the cleft area is essential before implant placement. In children whose lateral incisor space is preserved for future implant placement, the previously grafted area may show evidence of narrowing. An interval of several years between the bone graft and the implant placement is often inevitable if implant placement has been postponed until the patient has completed growth, which is the current guideline. The longer the interval, the greater the chance that bone will be insufficient for an implant, and that the previous graft will need additional bone. Patients who receive secondary bone grafts in the mixed dentition stage should have regrafting at 15 to 17 years of age, followed by implant placement within 4 months.

In young adolescent patients who complete orthodontic treatment, a Hawley retainer with plastic teeth will maintain the alignment and fill the empty spaces, thus providing good aesthetics and lip support (see Figs. 28-19, C and D). In the postadolescent period, the orthodontist determines when the patient's facial growth is complete. This is done by superimposing cephalometric radiographs obtained 6 months apart and comparing the changes over time (see Fig. 28-5, C). When completion of facial growth has been confirmed, the surgeon will regraft the cleft area if necessary and place implants. The prosthodontist completes the sequence by placing the final crown restorations.

CONCLUSION

A cleft lip and palate affect the development and position of the patient's jaws and teeth. Proper jaw and tooth anatomy is important for form and function. The orthodontist and surgeon work together and with the rest of the cleft team to develop an individualized treatment plan based on the patient's needs. The timing of this treatment depends on the patient's growth and development.

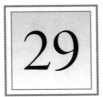

29

Alveolar Bone Grafting

Bernard J. Costello, Ramon L. Ruiz

KEY POINTS

○ Bone grafting to the upper jaw (alveolus and maxilla) is important for the health of the erupting permanent adult teeth.

○ In most patients, expansion of the upper jaw with an orthodontic expander is required before bone grafting.

○ The timing of the procedure is usually based on the developing teeth, as viewed on radiographs.

○ The bone graft is usually taken from the wing of the pelvis (hip bone) or other areas such as the skull, chin, or rib.

○ Bone usually needs to be placed into the cleft jaw area before the eruption of the developing teeth.

Despite successful lip repair and closure of the hard and soft palates during infancy, a residual opening and a bony cleft will usually persist in the alveolus (the bony ridge that houses the teeth). These residual gaps are most often treated by bone grafting.

The objectives of bone graft reconstruction of the cleft maxilla are to establish adequate bone for eruption of the permanent (adult) teeth in the area of the cleft, to close any residual gaps, to establish continuity of the jaw, and to improve the underlying support of the nose. For patients with a bilateral (two-sided) cleft lip and palate, bone grafting provides the added benefit of anchoring the often mobile premaxilla, the small central segment of bone in the upper jaw.

TIMING AND EVALUATION FOR BONE GRAFTING

Children with clefts of the lip will have a gap in the area of the upper jaw and teeth approximately 75% of the time. This area is most often left open intentionally through infancy and young childhood. However, it needs to be closed before the permanent teeth erupt into the cleft site. The timing of this procedure is based on the child's dental development and not the chronologic age (see Chapters 26 and 28). For this reason, radiographs are usually obtained when the child is 5 years of age to evaluate the developing teeth. Bone graft reconstruction of this site typically is performed during the mixed dentition stage, just before the eruption of the permanent canine and/or the permanent lateral incisor. This is known as secondary alveolar bone grafting and is performed during the mixed dentition stage, when the child is 6 to 10 years of age. During this stage of dental development, some of the baby teeth have been replaced by adult teeth (see Chapter 26). It is the most common and successful protocol worldwide.

A small number of teams prefer to perform the bone grafting procedure much earlier, before the eruption of any permanent teeth. This procedure is often called primary bone grafting. Most teams perform bone grafting later to prevent potential harm to the growth of the upper jaw. However, when bone grafting is performed just before the eruption of the adult teeth into the cleft area, the growth of the upper jaw is minimally affected.

Another option is gingivoperiosteoplasty, which closes the gap between the teeth with small, soft tissue flaps at the time of lip repair. This technique usually involves the use of an orthopedic molding device such as a nasoalveolar molding appliance (see Chapter 27). Some patients who have had this procedure develop bone at the cleft alveolar site, but many will also benefit from additional bone grafting of the nasal floor and/or the alveolar jaw bone later. This protocol is not widely accepted. Additional studies for earlier grafting procedures are ongoing.

Standard dental radiographs or a computed tomography (CT) scan is helpful for understanding the development of the permanent teeth to properly determine the timing of the grafting procedure. In most patients, bone grafting is performed when approximately half to three fourths of the roots of the teeth erupting at the cleft site is developed. Most children are 6 to 10 years of age at this developmental stage, but this varies considerably. Before surgery, it is often necessary to expand the upper jaw with an orthodontic expander. The exact timing is based on the dental age of the patient rather than the chronologic age. For example, in most patients, the central incisor (front tooth) is surrounded by adequate bone for proper and healthy eruption; in other patients, however, bone is insufficient, and this can usually be seen on the radiographs.

In most children, the permanent teeth erupt in the area around the cleft at 5 to 12 years of age. The teeth involved are typically the canine, the lateral incisor, and sometimes the central incisor (Fig. 29-1).

RECOMMENDED PROTOCOL

Once the surrounding teeth are appropriately developed, orthodontic expansion can begin. A specialized expander provided by an orthodontist, pediatric dentist, or dentist is used to widen the upper jaw to match the lower jaw shape. This minimizes the chance for a crossbite and the need for surgical expansion later. Widening the upper jaw early in this growth phase typically results in more stability and success than widening after growth is complete.

Most types of expanders are removed at the time of surgery or just before surgery. This will allow the surgeon to have complete control over design and elevation of the flaps and to close the residual holes or the unrepaired cleft behind the teeth. The expander can be replaced after the surgery, or another retention device, such as a wire or splint, can be used. For patients with bilateral clefts, the premaxilla must not interfere with the lower arch. Orthodontic/orthopedic techniques will be used to ensure that this segment is immobilized after the grafting procedure.

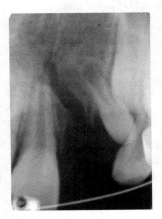

Fig. 29-1   A dental radiograph shows the cleft and the permanent teeth bordering the cleft. The erupting canine requires bone for its survival over the long term; therefore bone graft must be placed before eruption begins.

Motion of the premaxilla may cause problems with healing of the bone graft and soft tissues. A palatal splint, or a retainer-like device, may need to be placed after the graft is completed to minimize force on the premaxilla and to protect the graft from biting forces.

Primary (baby), supernumerary (extra), or nonrestorable (unfixable) teeth present in the cleft site may need to be extracted before grafting is performed. Adequate time for healing after extraction will be needed before the graft is placed. This provides additional gum tissue for alveolar repair at the time of the graft. Alternatively, teeth can be removed at the time of grafting.

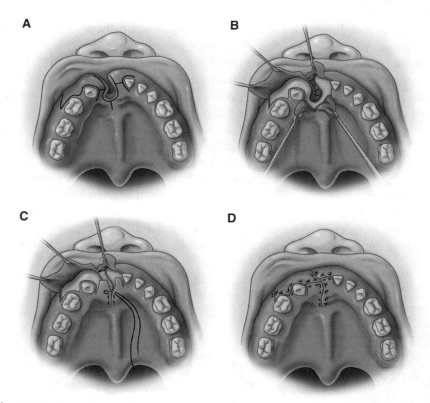

Fig. 29-2 Both a nasal-side closure and oral, or mouth, closure is completed with dissolvable stitches. Bone graft material is placed between these layers. One of the surgical goals is to provide near watertight closure of the nasal and oral sides of the cleft closure. **A,** Design of incisions for alveolar bone graft placement. **B,** Mucous membrane flaps lifted to expose the cleft in the bone. The nasal floor has been surgically repaired. **C,** The bone graft has been placed in the cleft before closure of the mucous membrane. **D,** Completed closure.

Incisions are made inside the mouth along the edges of the unrepaired cleft and the remaining openings (Fig. 29-2). The mucous membrane is usually closed in two layers with dissolvable stitches. One layer is that of the tissue in the mouth covering the teeth, and the other layer is that of the tissue inside the nasal cavity. Bone graft material is placed between these layers. One of the surgical goals is to provide near-watertight closure of the nasal side and oral side of the cleft closure.

Although bone graft can be taken from several sites, the iliac crest (part of the ilium, one of the bones of the pelvis) is used most often. A small incision is made just to the side of the prominence of the pelvic wing. Very limited work is required to obtain the necessary amount of bone marrow from a small area of the pelvis. Most patients have mild pain and can walk easily without assistance after the surgery. A small dressing may be placed after surgery.

POSTOPERATIVE CONSIDERATIONS

Swelling around the upper jaw is expected and typically peaks in several days. It is substantially resolved by 2 weeks after the procedure. Most patients have mild pain at the surgical site in the hip and can walk easily without assistance. Because of the mild discomfort, many children benefit from the use of pain medication for several days after surgery. Patients are usually restricted from playing sports or engaging in other strenuous activities for several weeks. A soft diet for the first few weeks after surgery is helpful to optimize healing. The upper teeth should not be brushed until the incisions have healed, but oral rinses may be used to maintain good oral hygiene and to keep the surgical site clean. If a fixed splint or retainer device is used postoperatively, this may be removed by the orthodontist or surgeon several weeks after the surgery. In some cases, a removable splint may be used until graft healing is complete. In all cases, the surgeon or orthodontist will obtain x-rays 3 to 6 months after surgery to assess the healing graft.

CONCLUSION

Bone grafting into the area of the upper jaw cleft is an important aspect of comprehensive cleft treatment. Bone is required for proper support and long-lasting health of the teeth that normally erupt into the cleft area.

Multispecialty coordinated planning for reconstruction of the cleft jaw and alveolar defects is an important part of comprehensive cleft care that is most often performed during mixed dentition. Careful timing that accounts for dental age and sound reconstructive methods based on scientific evidence provide safe and effective results. Surgeons and orthodontists should be mindful of the balance between the benefits of early intervention and the risk of growth restriction. Studies continue to emerge demonstrating the benefits of secondary bone grafting and those of other treatment options. When the principles outlined in this chapter are followed, predictable results can be expected.

30

Cleft Orthognathic Jaw Surgery

Stephen B. Baker, Jesse A. Goldstein

KEY POINTS

- Jaw surgery is performed to achieve proper facial dimensions and a normal occlusion (bite).

- Approximately 25% to 33% of patients with a history of cleft lip/palate have an underbite (class III occlusion) that will benefit from surgical correction.

- Jaw surgery is performed after facial growth is complete, at approximately 16 years of age for girls and 17 to 18 years of age for boys.

- X-ray images of the wrist or the face are evaluated to determine whether growth is complete.

- A child needs to have completed all orthodontic treatments (braces) before jaw surgery is performed.

- The upper jaw is almost always moved during surgery in patients with a history of cleft lip and/or palate. The lower jaw may need to be moved in some patients.

- Bone grafts may be necessary and are usually taken from the hip bone. This is similar to the bone graft procedure for an alveolar bone graft (see Chapter 29).

- The patient's jaw may be wired together for a brief period after the surgery. A liquid diet is required during this time.

- A period of orthodontic therapy will be necessary after surgery to fine-tune the occlusion and correct minor occlusal discrepancies such as an overbite or underbite.

The term orthognathic surgery is used to describe a surgery in which the upper jaw bone (maxilla), the lower jaw bone (mandible), or both are moved during surgery. The term orthognathic comes from the Greek words *orthos* (to straighten) and *gnathic* (related to the jaw). Typically, in a child with a cleft lip and/or palate, the upper jaw bone lacks projection. The goal in these patients is to bring the upper jaw into a proper bite or occlusion with the lower jaw bone. This will establish proper facial proportion and alignment of the top teeth with the bottom teeth to optimize function (breathing and chewing) and appearance. This chapter explains the process by which a child undergoing orthognathic surgery will be evaluated and describes the basic surgical procedures, postoperative care, and possible complications.

PREOPERATIVE CONSIDERATIONS

A cleft lip and/or palate can negatively affect facial growth. Midface retrusion (displacement of the upper jaw bone backward from its normal position) results from lack of growth of the upper jaw. Approximately 25% to 30% of children will have severe enough midface retrusion to benefit from orthognathic surgery. Surgeons describe malocclusion using a classification system. The most common malocclusion affecting children with a cleft is a class III occlusion. This is commonly known as an underbite.

The exact cause of midface retrusion is not known. Evidence shows that scarring from surgical procedures can result in inelasticity of the facial soft tissues, causing stunted facial growth. Although orthodontic procedures can hide the presence of mild class III malocclusions, orthognathic surgery is needed to correct severe class III deformities.

PREOPERATIVE EVALUATIONS AND TREATMENTS

Before surgery can be performed, the patient needs to be evaluated by several members of the cleft and/or craniofacial team. The surgeon uses all of the information obtained from these tests to develop the best surgical plan for the patient. This is discussed with the patient and parents.

Velopharyngeal Competence

Velopharyngeal competence (function of the soft palate and speech mechanism) is evaluated in patients before they have orthognathic surgery. The velopharyngeal mechanism is a series of muscles, nerves, and airways in the back of the throat responsible for transmission of sound energy and air pressure in the oral and nasal cavity (see Chapter 25). This mechanism is often affected in children with a cleft palate, resulting in hypernasal speech. In orthognathic surgery, the upper jaw is moved forward (maxillary advancement), pulling the soft palate away from the posterior pharyngeal wall (the wall at the back of the throat). This movement can have a negative effect on the proper functioning of the velopharyngeal mechanism. A preoperative evaluation of this mechanism by the team speech and language pathologist helps to predict possible effects of maxillary advancement on speech. Aggressive advancement of the upper jaw bone in a patient with borderline speech preoperatively can create or exacerbate velopharyngeal incompetence.

In patients who previously had a pharyngeal flap surgery to treat velopharyngeal incompetence, forward movement of the upper jaw bone will be more difficult. If the upper jaw bone needs to be moved forward a great distance in a patient who had a pharyngeal flap, the surgeon may want to move the lower jaw backward in the same surgery so that less upper jaw advancement is needed. (See Operative Procedure for more information about the surgical procedure.)

Dental Occlusion

Typically, preoperative orthodontic treatment is necessary to level, align, and decompensate the dental occlusion. The patient wears these braces for at least 6 to 12 months before surgery. Further orthodontic treatment may be necessary for 6 to 12 months after surgery, depending on the severity of the bite. The surgeon and/or orthodontist will obtain models of the patient's teeth if necessary to assess alignment. These aids are useful for determining the needed preoperative orthodontic treatment and the possible effects of surgery on dental alignment. Areas that have had alveolar bone grafts need to be examined to determine whether additional bone grafting will be necessary while the jaw surgery is being performed.

Physical Examination

Every patient has a thorough physical examination before surgery. Good oral hygiene and periodontal health are essential.

PREPARATION FOR SURGERY

Orthognathic surgery is generally performed as a hospital-based operation. The patient is admitted the day of the surgery. Parents can expect their child to be discharged one to several days later. The length of time in the hospital depends on the child's progress and the surgeon's preference.

Before surgery, the surgeon simulates the orthognatic surgery on models, and makes splints from these models. These are used to guide the placement of the jaws during surgery. The surgeon will review the surgical plan with the patient and family.

OPERATIVE PROCEDURE

To move the jaw bone to the ideal location, the surgeon performs a procedure known as an osteotomy. This involves making cuts in the bone to free it so that it can be moved. In a cleft patient with an underbite, cuts are made in the maxilla. In the ideal jaw location, the upper jaw fits together with the lower jaw to form the best occlusion and to restore proper facial proportion. The osteotomy in which the upper jaw is moved is called a *LeFort I osteotomy*.

In a LeFort I osteotomy, an incision is made inside the upper lip so that it is not visible. This allows access to the upper jaw bone so that it can be cut and moved. Once the upper jaw is mobile, it is moved into the best location, which the surgeon determined before surgery. A surgical splint is used to position the upper jaw in relation to the lower jaw. Titanium plates are placed, and screws are inserted to secure the upper jaw in its new position while the bone heals. Titanium does not set off airport alarms or interfere with MRI imaging that might be performed in the future. Titanium has never been shown to cause problems in the human body; therefore the plates and screws are not routinely removed.

Occasionally, the surgeon will notice a fistula, or hole in the palate, while performing a LeFort I osteotomy. This can be repaired during the surgery. Bone grafting may be necessary if the fistula involves the area where the teeth are located. Some patients have a short or borderline short soft palate. The surgeon might think that moving the maxilla forward to correct the entire underbite may cause hypernasality by advancing the soft palate, which is connected to the maxilla. In these patients, the surgeon might choose to correct the underbite with a combination of moving the upper jaw forward and the lower jaw backward. The operation to move the lower jaw backward is called a *mandibular osteotomy*.

To perform a mandibular osteotomy, the surgeon makes the incisions on the inside of the mouth. One of two types of mandibular osteotomy can be done to move the lower jaw backward: a sagittal split osteotomy or an inverted vertical ramus osteotomy. The sagittal split osteotomy is more common.

In a sagittal split osteotomy, incisions are made in the back of the mouth to expose the lower jaw bone. Cuts are made in the bone to divide it into three separate pieces: the right jaw joint segment (the right segment in the back or the right proximal segment), the left jaw joint segment (the left segment in the back or the left proximal segment), and the tooth-bearing piece (the front or distal segment). By separating the tooth-bearing segment from both of the jaw joints, it can be moved backward without altering the jaw joint (temporomandibular joint). As the tooth-bearing segment is moved backward, it overlaps the jaw joint piece on both sides. It is through this overlapping area of the bones that titanium screws are placed to secure the bones while they heal. The screws are not routinely removed. The only incisions that are visible after a sagittal split osteotomy are two small punctures on either side of the back of the jaw line. These are about 5 mm long and are used to drill the holes and place the screws for the fixation of the bone segments. These small wounds typically heal very well and are almost invisible after a year. Because screw fixation is used with the sagittal split, the upper and lower jaw either do not need to be secured to each other (*maxillomandibular fixation*), or they are secured to each other with elastic rubber bands or wires for a short period of time.

An inverted vertical ramus osteotomy is a less commonly performed alternative to a sagittal split osteotomy. The advantage of this procedure is that it is performed entirely through incisions inside of the patient's mouth. No scars develop on the skin. However, the disadvantage is that the patient's jaws need to be wired together for an extended period of time that ranges from 4 to 8 weeks, depending on the surgeon's preference. Because the incisions heal so well with the sagittal split osteotomy, and patients do not like having their jaws wired together for a prolonged period, the sagittal split osteotomy is the more popular technique for moving the jaw backward.

POSTOPERATIVE CARE

The patient is usually discharged from the hospital one to several days after the surgery. Major pain is not common. Most patients have mild discomfort that lasts for approximately 5 days. This is well managed with pain medication. Swelling, nasal and/or sinus congestion, and difficulty chewing food are common. Swelling is a result of unavoidable trauma from the surgery. Most swelling peaks over the course of 3 to 5 days. Most of the swelling resolves within 10 days, and the rest subsides within several months. Because the surgery involves the *maxillary sinuses,* congestion can result. Most patients have a week-long period of significant congestion. Saline (salt water) nasal sprays, decongestants, and cotton-tip applicators of diluted hydrogen peroxide for the nostrils can help to relieve symptoms. Congestion decreases as the swelling resolves. If maxillomandibular fixation was performed using elastic rubber bands or wires, these are usually removed within 2 weeks, but every case is different. The surgeon may have a reason to maintain the fixation for a longer period. When fixation is in place, a liquid diet is necessary. Typically, any liquid or food made into a liquid with a food processor is acceptable. Protein shakes and instant breakfasts, for example, are good forms of liquid nutrition. Soft solid foods will be approved by the surgeon when the patient is ready. Firm and solid foods should not be consumed for 10 weeks. Orthodontic treatment will be required to complete dental therapy.

COMPLICATIONS

Complications are rare. However, they can occur, and the patient and family need to be informed about them before surgery. Numbness of the upper cheeks and lower lip is to be expected immediately after jaw surgery. However, as the patient recovers, the sensation should return to normal. The sensory nerves of the lip and cheek can be permanently injured, causing permanent partial or total numbness of these areas after the surgery.

Postoperative bleeding is rare. The treatment can consist of nasal packing, or it might require another surgery in which the surgeon explores the area for the source and control the bleeding.

Infection is rare and can usually be treated with antibiotics. Occasionally, a revision surgery is necessary.

Jaw surgery is a major procedure. If the patient's bite is off by more than a few millimeters, another surgery may be necessary so that the teeth are in a better position in preparation for orthodontic treatment.

CONCLUSION

Skeletal growth typically ends between 14 and 16 years of age in girls and between 16 and 18 years of age in boys. Facial skeletal maturity can be determined through a series of facial X-ray images over time. The surgeon evaluates these images to identify cessation of growth. Alternatively, or along with facial images, the surgeon can examine X-rays of the patient's wrists for closure of the growth plates. If orthognathic surgery is performed before the facial skeleton reaches maturity, the likelihood of revision surgery will be increased because of unpredictable postoperative growth.

Afterword

The Power of Difference: Social and Cultural Issues Associated With Cleft and Craniofacial Conditions

Ronald P. Strauss, Stephanie E. Watkins, Barry L. Ramsey

KEY POINTS

○ *Stigma* associated with facial differences should be minimized or countered by a positive environment at home and in school.

○ Teasing and bullying should be recognized and addressed.

○ Facial differences should not be treated as facial inferiority.

○ Differences in appearance lead to broader perspectives, and this is to be celebrated.

Cleft lip, cleft palate, and craniofacial conditions can alter facial appearance and/or speech. A person whose facial appearance or speech is noticeably different from that of others often has different social experiences. These occur within a set of expectations and behaviors defined by the values and norms of the community. How a society or a community treats those who look different is a powerful indicator of fundamental values. Individuals with appearance and speech differences learn about social life—both positive and painful aspects—through the experience of being different. Thus it is worth considering how appearance and speech differences shape life experiences and success. Do such differences affect quality of life, social experience, school performance, dating, and employment? Appearance and differences often determine success and the answer to the question, "Who am I?" Yet many people with differences thrive despite negative experiences. This chapter examines social values, stigmas, teasing, and bullying. It offers practical guidance to parents, caregivers, and family members for enhancing resilience, health, and coping to promote positive life outcomes.

STIGMA AND FACIAL APPEARANCE

Being seen as different often implies being perceived by others as less than complete or limited. Negative social perceptions or attitudes, known as stigma, often suggest a moral judgment, usually a negative one. First impressions of a person's difference can lead to assumptions about how the person with the difference should act, behave, and be treated, including being ignored and discounted. The appearance of the face and speech differences are immediately noticed by others. The face is the initial focus and main target of attention when communicating with others. Facial appearance and attractiveness have a strong effect on psychological development and social relationships. This has been noted across societies and across various medical conditions that result in facial or speech differences.

Two primary categories of stigma relate to facial differences. An enacted stigma is a person's direct experience with the negative impressions of others, such as discrimination, rejection, teasing, bullying, and physical abuse. Family members and those close to the person with differences can also be affected by enacted stigma. Another category of stigma involves the self-evaluation and self-consciousness of the person with a facial difference—in other words, what the individual feels or perceives. This is known as an internalized stigma. It is the affected person's response to the negative feedback and reduced social perception.

TEASING AND BULLYING

Stigma, teasing, and bullying are evident in childhood and appear to peak during adolescence. Teasing and bullying are defined differently. Teasing is laughing at or criticizing someone in a way that is either friendly and good natured or cruel and unkind. It may be a way to provide another person with social feedback and moral guidance or it can be a means of control, but it is not negative. Bullying, however, is the use of power or intimidation to mistreat or threaten others. It can include verbal threats and/or physical attacks or pressure. Bullying is always a negative expression and can be deeply damaging to the person targeted.

By 7 years of age, children make judgments about physical attractiveness in peers. At this age, such judgments mirror adult perspectives. Specific strategies can be useful in responding to potential stigmatization, teasing, or bullying of children who have a facial difference. It is helpful to identify stigmas and be aware of the power of long-term stigmas. Teasing and bullying need to be discussed with health care providers, counselors, other family members, school officials and teachers, and religious leaders. Counseling and peer support may be effective. Group exercises and the development of sample scenarios allow children experiencing discrimination to rehearse appropriate responses when faced with negative social interactions.

SOCIAL ISSUES ASSOCIATED WITH HEALTH CARE

The birth of a child with a cleft or craniofacial condition is often a crisis in the life of the family. The family members are required to change their expectations of the child's needs and shift their focus on finding proper health care. The family will consider who can provide specialized health care for the infant, how health and feeding needs will be met, and how health costs will be covered. The family might need to plan for the future health, social, and developmental issues that can be associated with their child's condition. Other decisions often need to be made about the amount and timing of the health care and treatment provided. The family's beliefs about the condition, their ability to offer mutual support, and their norms regarding parental responsibility will guide decisions. Religious perspectives and ethnic or cultural values often provide the basis for making treatment decisions within the family. Social attitudes about children with facial differences can influence treatment choices and how families cope with the diagnosis and treatment.

HOW TO EFFECTIVELY WORK WITH HEALTH CARE PROVIDERS

Parents are often shocked when learning of their child's cleft or craniofacial condition. Prenatal ultrasound allows the visualization of many conditions and can provide the family and physicians with information about a child before birth. The prenatal diagnosis of a cleft provides parents time to educate themselves about future health care needs of their unborn child.

Often, the diagnosis is made at the time of delivery. This is an exciting and critical moment that is engraved into every parent's memory. Some parents have described physicians as overly negative or focused only on the child's limitations. Although parents and families should be informed of potential risks of a given condition, this information should be imparted with optimism.

Initially, the craniofacial team will focus on the child's cleft, appearance, and feeding issues. Soon thereafter, the focus will shift to broader issues; the cleft should not define the child. Craniofacial team members can help parents to envision a positive future for their child by initiating and encouraging a discussion about the child's potential.

The Cleft/Craniofacial Team

The fundamentals and benefits of team care are discussed in detail in Chapter 1. The cleft/craniofacial teams help parents to understand diagnostic information and to evaluate the health and needs of their child. Building a strong, trusting relationship with the team and its members is essential. The core principle of a cleft/craniofacial team is to provide high-quality, collaborative, patient-centered care. They also assist the family in managing stress.

After each team appointment, the team members will meet to discuss findings and to create a comprehensive treatment plan. The team should involve the family when planning the treatment options for the child. As the child matures and when appropriate, the child should be encouraged to participate in the treatment decisions.

Knowledge is power. This statement is particularly true of parents whose child has a cleft lip/palate. When working with a craniofacial team, the parents should bring written questions, ask questions as they arise, request clarification if needed, and take notes at appointments.

PROMOTING POSITIVITY

The following guidelines are helpful for parents of a child with a cleft or craniofacial condition:
- The child should be treated as normally as possible.
- The child should be encouraged to talk about the cleft or craniofacial condition when he or she is able to understand. The child's difference should not be a forbidden topic.
- When the child begins to look in a mirror and recognize that he or she is different, questions such as "Why was I born this way?" need to be answered honestly.
- Patience is essential when helping a child cope with anger and frustration about doctor appointments and surgeries.

- Photos of the child should be taken, especially at birth and before surgeries, but also throughout the child's life. The child might wish to review this history and share it with a future spouse or children. The parents often appreciate having a photo history to review their child's transformation.
- Parents should enjoy their child's awareness as it develops based on unique experiences with health care and school.

Parents generally thrive with information and support. Families often find it helpful to meet with other parents and families in similar circumstances. Parent and patient support networks are empowering and provide needed emotional and logistical support for parents and siblings.

Child patients can benefit from support networks such as the following:
- Health care professionals: Team members, including social workers, psychologists, and nurses, who provide emotional support to parents and the child.
- Internet: Much information is available on the Internet, but caution should be used when reading what is posted on websites. Cleft/craniofacial team members can help parents by guiding their search for information, ensuring the data are accurate, and interpreting information.
- School systems: A discussion with teachers and counselors about the child's cleft/craniofacial condition can be helpful. Teachers can provide parents with valuable information and referral to other services available in the school system (for example, speech-language therapy) (see Chapter 13).

EDUCATE AND EMPOWER

Children with differences, their parents, other family members, and friends should be informed as much as possible about the condition. The following statements explain ways in which parents can educate and empower their child.
- Parents can educate their child and instill the strength to embrace the facial difference. Comeback lines can be taught and rehearsed. The child can use these when being teased or bullied about his or her craniofacial condition. As the child matures into adulthood, parents should encourage their child to seek additional medical advice such as genetic counseling to help understand the chance of having a child with a cleft.
- Parents should educate their family and friends about their child's difference. They will want to understand the condition and can be a source of support during challenging times such as surgeries.

- Parents should educate their child's teachers and counselors about their child's condition. Having an open line of communication with them can help parents understand what is happening at school, especially if their child has specific concerns with hearing, vision, speech, bullying, or teasing.
- Parents should not give up on their dreams. They should keep their dreams alive for their child and believe in the child's ability to fulfill them. By creating an environment of optimism and positivity, parents help their child thrive.

CONCLUSION

Children with a facial difference have unique identities with something special to add to the community. This view can profoundly alter how children with facial or speech differences are treated in social situations and understood by health professionals. These children should not be expected to change or hide themselves; rather, they can be encouraged to share their unique perspectives and contributions with others. If this is achieved, then people with facial difference—or any other form of difference—will be empowered to determine their own needs, define their life path, and make decisions about their future without the fear of judgment, pressures to conform, and stigma.

Appendix 1

Timeline of Care

TIMELINE OF COMPREHENSIVE CLEFT CARE

Fig. A-1 is a basic guide to the timing of procedures for treating patients with an orofacial cleft. Approximate times are provided; timing is based on individual growth and development. The exact timing and nature of the procedures performed varies between treatment centers.

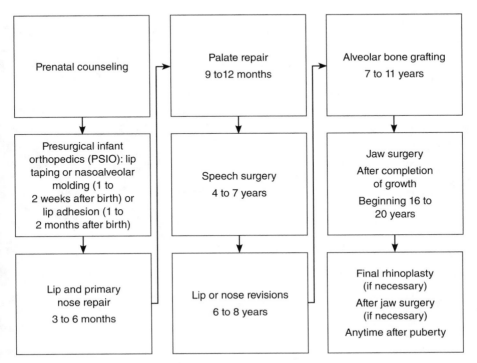

Fig. A-1   Timing of procedures for cleft-affected patients.

Appendix 2

Parameters of Care

This appendix summarizes the American Cleft Palate-Craniofacial Association's *Parameters for Evaluation and Treatment of Patients With Cleft Lip/Palate or Other Craniofacial Anomalies,* which is available at *http://www.acpa-cpf.org/uploads/site/ Parameters_Rev_2009.pdf.*

INTERDISCIPLINARY TEAMS

- Cleft and craniofacial teams are composed of individuals specializing in many fields, most frequently: hearing; genetic counseling; nursing; dentistry and orthodontics; pediatric medicine; ear, nose, and throat medicine; plastic surgery; psychology; social work; and speech.
- The team members work together to provide expertise and to develop a comprehensive integrated plan to optimize patient outcomes with the most efficient use of resources and family time.

NEONATAL PERIOD AND INFANCY

- A child born with a cleft should be evaluated by the cleft and craniofacial team during the first few days of life, with regularly scheduled appointments thereafter.
- The team should closely monitor the infant's growth and development and ensure that he or she is seen by all necessary members of the team at each visit.

LONGITUDINAL EVALUATION AND TREATMENT

- Audiologic care: Hearing should be tested within the first 3 months of life. A treatment plan should be created and customized to meet each patient's needs (for example, the need for ear tubes and treatment of hearing loss).

- Cleft lip/palate surgery: A cleft lip is generally repaired when the child is 3 to 6 months of age, and a cleft palate is repaired when the child is 9 to 12 months of age. Additional procedures and revisions will probably be required later in life.
- Maxillofacial surgery: Jaw surgery may be required to correct the patient's bite and facial proportions once the face has stopped growing (late adolescence to early adulthood).
- Dental care: A dedicated pediatric dentist is best suited to provide the often complex dental care necessary in patients with a cleft.
- Genetic services: Genetic counselors provide information regarding the patient's diagnosis (clefts might be associated with genetic conditions), including the risk of having a child with a cleft and how the genetic condition may affect the patient throughout life.
- Nursing care: Nurses play an essential role in educating families regarding the specialized care a child with a cleft may require and in serving as an interface for the patient, the family, and members of the cleft team.
- Otolaryngologic (ear, nose, and throat [ENT]) care: The ear, nose, and throat must be carefully monitored and treated in patients with a cleft, because these areas are frequently affected by associated issues (for example, ear infections or hearing difficulties in children with a cleft palate).
- Pediatric care: The pediatrician provides general medical care, coordinates specialty care as outlined in the treatment plan developed by the cleft team, and ensures that the child is healthy enough to undergo any planned operations.
- Psychological and social services: Social workers, psychologists, and psychiatrists play a key role in ensuring the emotional health of the child with a cleft and his or her family. Social workers help families overcome obstacles to receiving care prescribed by the cleft team (for example, financial and travel-related difficulties).
- Speech-language pathology services: Children with a cleft palate have a high risk of developing speech and language problems. Speech pathologists diagnose these problems, may recommend surgery and/or speech therapy, and provide speech therapy when needed.
- Quality management: Cleft team quality of care is monitored by assessing patient progress over time, reviewing the success of treatment strategies as defined by specific outcomes, and adapting treatment strategies when goals are not met.
- Revisions of clinical practices: The diagnosis and treatment practices outlined in this book will change as medical knowledge and technology improve over time. It is the responsibility of the cleft and craniofacial teams to monitor the results of their treatment protocols and to revise their clinical practices to provide the highest quality, state-of-the-art care.

Glossary

22q11.2 deletion syndrome   A genetic disorder caused by absence of a small piece of genetic material on chromosome 22. Also known as velocardiofacial syndrome or DiGeorge syndrome, the disorder may present with congenital heart disease, immunological abnormalities, speech and learning problems, and a characteristic facial appearance.

acid reflux   Flow of acidic fluid from the stomach back into the esophagus, the tube connecting the mouth to the stomach.

adenoid   A mass of lymphoid tissue on the back of the throat, behind the palate. Part of the body's immune system, the adenoid may be removed without harm to immune function.

adenoidectomy   Surgical removal of the adenoid.

alar base   The portion of the nostril that attaches to the upper lip.

alveolus   The ridge of bone, covered by the gums, that houses the teeth.

amniocentesis   Prenatal test to diagnose genetic differences in the fetus. The test involves sampling a small amount of amniotic fluid from the sac around the fetus.

anterior crossbite   Malocclusion in which the front teeth of the upper jaw are positioned behind those of the lower jaw.

apnea   A pause in breathing during sleep.

apnea-hypopnea index   A measure of the severity of apnea, represented by the number of pauses in breathing per hour of sleep.

apraxia   A speech disorder characterized by abnormal planning of speech movements by the brain.

articulation   The movement and placement of the lips, tongue, teeth, and jaws during the production of speech.

aspiration   The abnormal passage of stomach contents into the airway.

audiologist   Medical professional who specializes in the diagnosis and management of hearing disorders.

auditory brainstem response (ABR)   A hearing test, often performed after a newborn fails an initial hearing screen, that measures the response of the nervous system to sounds.

aural atresia   Underdevelopment of the ear canal and middle ear; usually present with microtia.

bifid uvula   A uvula that is split in two parts, often associated with submucosal cleft palate.

bilateral cleft lip   A cleft that involves both sides of the upper lip.

biopsychosocial assessment   Determining the patient's medical, emotional, and relationship issues.

bone conduction   Transmission of sounds through vibration of the bone of the skull.

buccal sulcus   Valley of mucosa-covered soft tissue between the gingiva and the lip.

canine substitution   Replacement of a missing lateral incisor through the orthodontic movement of the canine tooth into its position.

caries   Dental cavities.

central sleep apnea   A pause in breathing caused by a failure of the brain to signal the muscles of respiration.

cephalometric radiograph   A standardized x-ray of the head, demonstrating the facial bones, the teeth, and their relationship to one another.

chorionic villus sampling   A prenatal test to determine genetic disorders in the fetus. It involves obtaining a sample of placental tissue.

chromosome   A structure within the cell that contains genetic material.

cleft lip   A birth defect characterized by a split in one or both sides of the upper lip.

cleft lip and nose adhesion   Surgical procedure in which the two parts of the cleft lip are joined together with sutures.

cleft palate   A birth defect characterized by a split in the roof of the mouth.

cochlea   Spiral-shaped hearing organ of the inner ear.

cochlear implant   An implanted electronic medical device that helps to provide sound signals to the brain when the cochlea is damaged.

columella   The strip of skin extending from the tip of the nose to the upper lip and separating the nostrils.

compensatory misarticulation   An abnormal pattern of articulation associated with velopharyngeal dysfunction or insufficiency.

complete cleft lip   A cleft that extends completely through the upper lip and into the nose.

conductive hearing loss   Hearing loss resulting from a problem in the conduction of sound waves through the outer ear, the eardrum, and the bones of the middle ear.

continuous positive airway pressure (CPAP)   A therapy for sleep apnea that involves gently blowing air through the nose or through the mouth and nose using a facemask.

CPAP titration study   Sleep study in which the patient wears a continuous positive airway pressure mask to determine the amount of air pressure that is required to open the child's airway with the device.

craniofacial   Related to or involving the cranium (skull) and face.

craniomaxillofacial surgery   Surgical procedure involving the bones and soft tissues of the face and skull.

crossbite   Malocclusion in which the upper teeth are positioned behind the lower teeth.

cyanosis   Blue skin color, representing a low blood oxygen level.

dentin   The hard tissue that is covered by the enamel of the teeth.

dentition   The teeth.

desaturation   Decrease in oxygen in the blood.

distraction osteogenesis   Surgical procedure in which two segments of bone are slowly moved apart, allowing new bone to form in the gap.

dysarthria   A speech disorder caused by impaired movement of the muscles responsible for speech production.

eardrum   The "tympanic membrane"; a thin filament that separates the outer ear from the inner ear.

early intervention   A system providing for assessment and therapy services for young children (usually birth to age 3 years) to facilitate normal development.

ectopic teeth   Teeth that have erupted into an improper location.

enamel   The hard outer layer of the teeth.

ENT surgeon   Also called an otolaryngologist, a physician specializing in disorders of the ear, nose, and throat.

Eustachian tube   Tube that connects the middle ear to the back of the throat. It is necessary to maintain normal aeration of the middle ear.

Eustachian tube dysfunction   Inadequate opening of the Eustachian tube (can be caused by incorrectly formed muscles associated with a cleft palate). This can lead to poor drainage and resulting infections of the middle ear.

external pacing   Removing the nipple from the infant's mouth to decrease the flow of milk or formula until the infant can catch a breath.

extraoral   Outside the mouth.

Family and Medical Leave Act (FMLA)   Law that entitles eligible employees to take unpaid, job-protected leave for specified family and medical reasons while maintaining health care benefits.

fistula   Abnormal passage between two spaces. An abnormal passage between the mouth and nose through the palate is termed an *oronasal fistula*.

Furlow palatoplasty   A technique of palate repair that closes the palate in a zig-zag fashion (see *Z-plasty*).

gene   A molecule made of DNA that functions as the basic unit of heredity. Genes contain information that determines the characteristics in children that will be passed on to them from their parents.

genetic counselor   A health professional with specialized training in medical genetics and counseling.

geneticist   A physician that specializes in the science of human genetics.

gingiva   The soft tissue of the gums.

gingivoperiosteoplasty   A surgical procedure to repair the gums at the site of a cleft in the alveolus. Primary gingivoperiosteoplasty refers to this procedure when it is performed at the time of cleft lip repair.

glossoptosis   Posterior (backward) displacement of the tongue, often leading to upper airway obstruction. One of the features of Pierre Robin sequence.

Goldenhaar syndrome   Rare condition is present at birth. The infant has incomplete development of the ears, nose, soft palate, lips, and jaw.

hard palate   Front portion of the roof of the mouth, made up of mucous membrane covering bone.

Hawley retainer   Removable, custom-made intraoral appliance made of acrylic and wires that helps to maintain the position of the teeth and the shape of the dental arch.

hypernasality   Excessive sound, or resonance, coming through the nose during speech.

hypertrophic scar   An abnormal scar that is thickened, firm, and reddened.

hyponasality   Too little sound, or resonance, coming through the nose during speech.

hypopnea   Abnormally slow or shallow breathing.

incisive foramen   An opening in the palatal bone behind the front teeth, located at the junction of the premaxilla and the palatine bones. This is a normal structure through which nerves and blood vessels pass.

incomplete cleft lip   A cleft that passes partially through the upper lip, not extending into the nose.

Individual Education Plan (IEP)   A written education plan designed to meet a child's unique learning issues, outlining specific educational goals.

Individual Family Service Plan (IFSP)   A written plan providing for early intervention services that a child and family will receive.

Individuals With Disabilities Education Act   A federal law that mandates early intervention services for all children with disabilities or developmental delays.

inner ear   The innermost part of the ear, responsible for sound transduction and balance. It is made up of the cochlea (which senses sound) and the semicircular canals (which control balance).

intraoral   Inside the mouth.

intravelar veloplasty   Surgical repair of the levator muscles within the soft palate.

Klippel-Feil syndrome   Congenital bone disorder characterized by fusion of two or more spinal bones in the neck.

language   The acquisition and use of a system of communication that employs sounds and/or symbols.

larynx   The voice box, containing the vocal cords.

Latham device   A pin-retained, screw-activated, intraoral device used to bring the segments of the palate closer together before cleft repair.

LeFort I osteotomy   A surgical procedure in which the upper jaw is cut and moved forward to normalize the relationship between the upper and lower jaws.

levator veli palatini   Also referred to as the *levator*, the muscle that is primarily responsible for movement of the palate during speech.

lip and nose adhesion   A preliminary partial repair of a cleft lip, often used in wide clefts as an alternative to presurgical orthopedics.

lymphoid tissue   Tissue such as the tonsils and adenoids that functions as part of the body's immune system. The tonsils and adenoids can be removed without harm to the immune system.

malignant hyperthermia   Serious reaction to anesthesia that is characterized by high fever, redness, and muscle stiffness.

malocclusion   Abnormal relationship between the teeth of the upper and lower jaws.

Manchester repair   A method of cleft lip repair (no longer commonly used) that discards very little tissue from the prolabium and includes an anterior (in the front) cleft palate repair with the lip repair.

mandible   The lower jaw.

mandibular osteotomy   Surgery in which a cut is made in the lower jaw so that it can be moved forward.

maxilla   The upper jaw.

maxillary sinuses   Air-filled space in the upper jaw bone that connects with the nose.

maxillomandibular fixation   Fastening of the upper jaw to the lower jaw to stabilize these structures during healing.

micrognathia   A condition in which the lower jaw is abnormally small.

microtia   A condition characterized by a small, malformed outer ear.

middle ear   The part of the ear behind the eardrum, responsible for the conversion of sound energy into mechanical energy. It consists of the eardrum itself and the hollow space behind the eardrum. The middle ear contains three small bones, or *ossicles*, that transfer the vibrations of the eardrum to the inner ear.

middle-ear disease   Infection (often beginning with fluid collection) or other disturbance in the function of the portion of the ear between the outer ear and the inner ear. May lead to hearing loss if not prevented or treated.

middle-ear effusion   An abnormal accumulation of fluid or mucous in the middle ear.

midface hypoplasia   A condition characterized by abnormally reduced growth of the upper jaw and cheekbones.

mucous membrane   The tissue lining the interior of the mouth and nose.

multiview videofluoroscopy   A technique used to assess function of the palate using a video x-ray of the palate during speech.

myringotomy   A surgical procedure to create an incision in the eardrum, usually to place tympanostomy tubes.

Nager syndrome   Rare condition present at birth that mainly affects the hands, arms, and face. Hearing ability is often affected.

nasalance   A measure of the degree of velopharyngeal opening during speech, calculated as the ratio of sound energy coming through the nose to that coming through the mouth.

nasal septum   Partition that separates the two sides of the nasal airway, composed of bone and cartilage covered by mucous membrane.

nasal splint/nasal stent   A silicone appliance placed in the nose, used to maintain the shape of the nose after cleft repair.

nasendoscopy   A procedure in which a flexible fiberoptic camera is passed through the nose to examine the function of the palate during speech.

nasoalveolar molding (NAM)   A technique of presurgical orthopedics, used to narrow the cleft and to improve the shape of the nose before surgical repair.

nasometer   An instrument used to measure nasalance.

nasopharyngoscopy   See *nasendoscopy.*

neonatal teeth   Small teeth present at or shortly after birth.

obstructive sleep apnea   A pause in breathing caused by a narrowing or blockage of the airway.

occlusion   Relationship between the upper and lower teeth.

ophthalmologist   A physician who specializes in the diagnosis and management of disorders of the eye.

oral surgeon   A physician who specializes in surgery of the teeth and jaws.

orofacial cleft   A gap or split in the structures of the face and/or jaws, most commonly affecting the lip, nose, and palate.

oronasal fistula   An opening through the palate that connects the mouth and the nose.

orthodontist   A dental professional who specializes in straightening and aligning the teeth.

orthognathic surgery   Surgical procedure performed to correct the position of the upper and/or lower jaws.

ossicles   The small bones in the middle ear that amplify the vibrations of the ear drum and transmit sound energy to the inner ear.

otoacoustic emissions   First-line hearing screening performed at birth.

otolaryngologist   See *ENT surgeon.*

oval window   An opening between the middle and inner ear through which the stapes transmits vibrations.

palate   The roof of the mouth, composed of the hard palate and soft palate.

palatoplasty   Surgical procedure to repair a cleft palate.

panoramic radiograph   Dental x-ray displaying the upper and lower jaws and teeth.

percuss   To tap with the palm of the hand. This is done to an infant's back to improve airflow in the lungs.

permanent (secondary) teeth   The adult teeth.

pharyngeal flap   A surgical procedure for the treatment of velopharyngeal dysfunction in which a small piece of tissue from the back of the throat is attached to the soft palate.

pharyngeal walls   The mucosal/muscular structures that make up the back and sides of the throat (pharynx).

pharynx   The throat.

philtrum   The central, normally dimpled portion of the upper lip.

Pierre Robin sequence   A congenital condition in which the infant has a small lower jaw (micrognathia), a tongue that falls back into the upper airway (glossoptosis), and difficulty breathing (apnea).

pinna   Outer part of the ear.

plastic surgeon   A physician who specializes in the surgical restoration of form and function.

polysomnogram   Also called a "sleep study," a medical test used to diagnose abnormal sleep patterns and breathing problems during sleep.

pontic   "Dummy" tooth placed on retainers, implants, and bridges to replace missing teeth, also known as a prosthetic tooth.

posterior crossbite   Malocclusion in which the back teeth of the upper jaw are positioned behind or inside of the teeth of the lower jaw.

premaxilla   The segment of bone in the central upper jaw that normally contains the four upper incisors.

prenatal   Before birth.

pressure-equalizing (PE) tube   Also known as a tympanostomy or myringotomy tube, a small tube placed in the eardrum to allow fluid to drain from the middle ear and to keep the middle ear aerated.

presurgical infant orthopedics   Any of several methods used to align the segments of the palate and gums and to improve the shape of the lip and nose before cleft repair.

primary teeth   The baby teeth.

proclination   Forward tipping of the teeth.

prolabium   The central portion of the upper lip, attached to the premaxilla, in a child with a bilateral cleft lip.

prone positioning   Positioning in which an infant is lying facedown. Often used in the management of infants with Pierre Robin sequence.

prosthodontist   A dental professional specializing in the prosthetic restoration or replacement of teeth.

psychologist   A mental health professional specializing in the evaluation and treatment of behavioral and mental disorders.

psychosocial   Relating to those concepts that involve psychological processes and social function.

radiograph   An x-ray.

REM sleep   One of the stages of sleep, characterized by rapid eye movements. It is the stage of sleep when dreaming occurs.

resonance   An acoustical attribute of speech, related to the modification of sound vibrations as they pass from the vocal cords through the vocal tract.

retroclination   Backward tipping of the teeth.

retrusion   Condition in which a structure is behind its normal position.

rhinoplasty   Surgery to alter the form and/or function of the nose.

self-concept   The collection of beliefs that one develops about oneself.

sensorineuronal hearing loss   Hearing loss that is the result of a problem in the inner ear or in the nerve pathway from the inner ear to the brain.

serum bicarbonate   A component in the blood that, when elevated, can indicate that a patient has obstructive sleep apnea.

Simonart's band   Small band of tissue at the base of the nostril that connects the lip segments together in a cleft lip.

sleep apnea   A condition characterized by pauses in breathing during sleep.

sleep study   See *polysomnogram*.

social worker   A professional who specializes in supporting children and families in need of assistance through counseling, advocacy, education, crisis intervention, and access to available resources.

soft palate   The back portion of the palate, composed of mucous membrane covering muscle.

special education   The specialized practice of educating children and adults with learning disabilities and/or developmental delays in a manner that addresses their unique differences and needs.

speech-language pathologist   A professional specializing in communication (and sometimes feeding) disorders.

sphincter pharyngoplasty   A surgical technique for the treatment of velopharyngeal dysfunction in which tissue from behind the tonsils is rearranged to narrow the opening of the velopharyngeal valve.

Stickler syndrome   A group of genetic conditions commonly associated with cleft palate and Pierre Robin sequence. Other features include a characteristic facial appearance, visual abnormalities, hearing loss, and joint problems.

stigma   A set of negative beliefs about a person or group held by others in society.

submucous cleft palate   A cleft of the palate characterized by a split in the interior muscles of the soft palate without disruption of the overlying mucous membrane.

supernumerary teeth   Extra teeth.

supine position   Position in which a person is lying on the back.

syndrome   A group of differences that appear together and that collectively characterize a specific disease or medical condition.

tidal volume   Depth of breathing.

Title V Maternal and Child Health Program   A state-federal partnership enacted in 1935 as part of the Social Security Act. It provides funding to help ensure the health of women, infants, and children.

tongue-lip adhesion   A surgical procedure in which the tip of the tongue is temporarily attached to the inside of the lower lip. The technique is sometimes used for the treatment of glossoptosis and upper airway obstruction in infants with Pierre Robin sequence.

tonsillectomy   Surgical removal of the tonsils.

tonsils   Paired lymphoid organs located on either side of the back of the throat.

Treacher Collins syndrome   Condition present at birth that causes various degrees of underdeveloped facial bones. Some of these children have a cleft palate.

tympanic membrane   The eardrum.

tympanometry   Test that evaluates eardrum mobility in response to changes in air pressure presented through the ear canal.

tympanostomy tube   Ventilation tube (also known as a pressure-equalization tube or PE tube) that is surgically placed into the eardrum to maintain aeration in the middle ear.

unilateral cleft lip   A cleft that involves one side of the upper lip.

uvula   Small, fingerlike projection of soft tissue at the back of the soft palate.

velocardiofacial syndrome   Congenital condition that causes differences in the palate, heart, and kidneys and can affect the immune system, speech, and learning. Also known as 22q11.2 deletion syndrome.

velopharyngeal dysfunction (VPD)   Also called velopharyngeal incompetence or velopharyngeal insufficiency (VPI), a condition in which the velopharynx does not function properly during speech, allowing for abnormal escape of air through the nose.

velopharyngeal insufficiency   See *velopharyngeal dysfunction (VPD)*.

velopharynx   That area of the anatomy, defined by the back of the soft palate and the walls of the pharynx, responsible for controlling the flow of air through the mouth and nose during speech.

velum   The soft palate.

vestibular stenosis   Narrowing of the nasal passage just inside the nostril, usually caused by scarring.

videofluoroscopy   See *multiview videofluoroscopy*.

vomer   Bone within the nasal septum. The mucous membrane covering the vomer is often used to close the floor of the nose during cleft palate repair.

Z-plasty   Method of tissue rearrangement in which a Z-shaped incision is made and the resulting triangles are transposed. In the Furlow cleft palate repair, this technique is used to lengthen the soft palate.

Credits

Chapter 4
Figs. 4-1 through 4-4   Courtesy of Dr. Joseph E. Losee, Children's Hospital of Pittsburgh.

Fig. 4-5   From Tewfik TL, Meyers AD, Kanaan A, et al. Cleft lip and palate and mouth and pharynx deformities. Available at *http://emedicine.medscape.com/article/837347-overview.*

Fig. 4-6   From Eppley BL, van Aalst JA, Robey A, et al. The spectrum of orofacial clefting. Plast Reconstr Surg 115:101e-114e, 2005.

Chapter 7
Fig. 7-4   Courtesy of Mary Spano.

Chapter 28
Fig. 28-1   Courtesy of Jack Lude, MD, Nationwide Children's Hospital, Columbus, Ohio.

Fig. 28-3   From Vig KW, Mercado AM. The orthodontist's role in a cleft palate–craniofacial team. In Graber TM, Vanarsdall RL, Vig KWL, eds. Orthodontics: Current Principles and Techniques, ed 5. Philadelphia, 2012; with kind permission from Elsevier, Inc.

Figs. 28-4 through 28-6; Fig. 28-11   Reprinted from Vig KWL, Mercado AM. The orthodontist's role in a cleft palate–craniofacial team. In Graber TM, Vanarsdall RL, Vig KWL, eds. Orthodontics: Current Principles and Techniques, ed 5. Philadelphia, 2012; with kind permission from Elsevier, Inc.

Index

Index **343**

testing considerations for very young children in, 108-109
with 22q11.2 deletion syndrome, 112-113
variables affecting, 106
Elbow splints
after cleft lip repair, 76
after cleft palate repair, 79
after unilateral cleft lip and nose repair, 205
Electrocardiogram, 184
Electroencephalogram, 178, 179, 184
Elementary school assessments by social worker, 123-124
Emergence delirium, 192
Emotional issues after cleft lip repair, 77
Employee Retirement Income Security Act (1974), 19
Empowerment, 320-321
Enacted stigma, 318
Enamel defects, 258
Endolymphatic sac, 156
ENT (ear, nose, and throat) care, parameters of care for, 326
Eruption of primary teeth, 257-258
Eustachian tube, 148, 149, 156
Eustachian tube dysfunction, 130, 149-150
treatment for, 150-151
Exhalation, 132
Expansion device, 280-281, 286, 287, 305-306
External pacing, 67

F

Face mask therapy, 280-281
Facial appearance, 318
Facial grimacing, 140
Family constellation, assessment of, 117-118
Family and Medical Leave Act (FMLA, 1993), 117, 121
Family as team members, 12-13
Fasting before surgery, 190
Feeding, 65-75
and acid reflux, 74
of adopted cleft-affected child, 27-29
after alveolar bone grafting, 80
assisted, 256
breast, 71-73
burping after, 67
choking during, 74
after cleft lip repair, 75-76
after cleft palate repair, 78
distress and discomfort during, 66
external pacing of, 67
feeding bottles and nipples for, 68-71
frequency of, 74
frequently asked questions about, 73-75
insurance coverage for, 66

length of, 66, 74
with nasoalveolar molding therapy, 62-63, 272
positioning for, 66, 67, 71-72
prenatal consultation on, 55
principles and techniques for, 65-66
after secondary palatal surgery, 81
social worker assessment of, 121
of solid foods, 74-75
step-by-step instructions for, 66-67
of toddler, 87
video on, 66
volume of, 66, 73
and weight gain, 66
Feeding bottles, 68-71
Feeding and swallowing therapy, 138
Fetal echocardiography, 43
Fetal hydantoin (Dilantin) syndrome, 45
Fetal magnetic resonance imaging (MRI), 42, 43
Financial situation, assessment of, 117
Fistula, 135, 140, 230, 284
501(c)(3) nonprofit organizations, advocacy by, 15-16
504 plans, 20
Fluency disorder, 141
Fluoride therapy, 260
FMLA (Family and Medical Leave Act, 1993), 117, 121
Furlow double-opposing Z-plasty
for cleft palate repair, 227-229
potential complications of, 248
for submucous cleft palate, 220-221
for velopharyngeal dysfunction, 246, 247-248

G

Gasping, 181
Gastroesophageal reflux, 74
Gene(s), 43
Gene mutations, 44-45
Genetic counseling
for adolescent, 91
parameters of care for, 326
postnatal, 48
preconception, 47-48
prenatal, 41-47
Genetic mutation, 44
Genetic testing
prenatal, 43-47
for submucous cleft palate, 218
Genetically based classification systems, 40
Genetics evaluation for Pierre Robin sequence, 172
Gestures, 110
Gingival inflammation, 260
Gingivoperiosteoplasty, 230, 304